About Globetrotter

When illness or injury strikes while traveling, an accurate diagnosis and prompt medical attention are essential to a good outcome. Across the world physicians ask many relevant questions while evaluating a patient's medical problem. Good communication is necessary in diagnosing potentially life-threatening emergencies such as heart attack, stroke, appendicitis, shock, convulsions, loss of blood, head trauma, and severe infection.

In *The Globetrotter's Pocket Doc*, these urgent situations are covered as well as other major and minor illnesses and injuries. This book contains statements, prepared by a physician and reviewed by a panel of Board Certified physicians and nurses, which pertain to the symptoms the patient may be experiencing. Beside each entry is a checkbox along with the French translation. By checking the appropriate symptom, the patient can impart information regarding his or her condition prior to treatment.

Medical history forms for all travelers—infants, children, and adults—are also included. These are to be completed prior to travel. This medical history, along with detailed information on the traveler's current health problems, arm the physician with the necessary information to make an accurate diagnosis and choose the appropriate treatment.

Also included in *The Globetrotter's Pocket Doc*
- A broad list of prescription and nonprescription drugs with their generic names and French translation and the condition each medication is designed to treat
- Metric conversion charts for weight and temperature
- A visual field diagram to assist in diagnosing eye problems
- Anatomic diagrams to help the patient indicate the location of the medical condition, pain, or injury that has been sustained
- Information on outpatient care for a variety of medical conditions that do not require treatment by healthcare providers

Globetrotter's Pocket Doc

English/French

Globetrotter's Pocket Doc

An International Medical Translator

English/French

Jonathan E. Jensen, MD, FACP

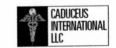

Caduceus International, LLC

P.O. Box 144
Hygiene, CO 80533

Globetrotter's Pocket Doc: An International Medical Translator

© 2004 Jonathan E. Jensen

Jensen, Jonathan E.
  An international medical translator. French /
[Jonathan E. Jensen].
  p. cm. -- (Globetrotters's pocket doc series)
  Includes index
  LCCN 2002090856
  ISBN 0-9718056-4-4

  1. Medicine--Terminology. 2. French language--
Conversation and phrase books--English. 3. french
language--Conversation and phrase books (for medical
personnel)   I. Title.

R123.J46 2004   610'.14
                           QB103-200871

Cover and interior design: Robert Aulicino

ACKNOWLEDGMENTS

I WANT TO ACKNOWLEDGE NUMEROUS PERSONS WHO HAVE FILLED MY life and work. I particularly want to thank my wife Judy and my children Jonathan and Johanna, all of whom have been gracious enough to allow me to spend the time researching and writing this book. Judy has given me the inspiration required to pursue this endeavor even when it meant a great deal of time away from the rest of my wonderful family. Her input and backup have made this book possible. It is a gift I will cherish from the most important person in my life.

To the rest of my immediate family, I must give due appreciation to my brother Christopher and sister-in-law Cheryl (outstanding tolerance to numerous phone calls), my sister Johanna (outstanding tolerance to almost anything), and most importantly to my parents, Phoebe and Wallace Jensen, without whom none of me would be possible. My father, Wallace N. Jensen, MD MACP, instilled in me a determination to treat patients with care and respect while putting second all other concerns. He has taught me medicine through compassion and understanding—a gift I will carry and reference for the rest of my life.

Special thanks go to Dr. John and Nina Sessions of Chapel Hill, North Carolina who must be mentioned because of their unswerving support throughout of my life. This is a debt I can never repay but hope to pass on to others.

Professionally, I am grateful for my professors and colleagues with whom I have worked through the years at Albany Medical Center in Albany, New York; Yale University in New Haven, Connecticut; The Cleveland Clinic Florida in Ft. Lauderdale, Florida; University of Colorado Health Sciences Center in Denver, Colorado; and to Dr. Drew Geer (emergency MD extraordinaire) for his direction and additional writing.

Others who have worked on this text are numerous. I am particularly indebted to Mary Embree of Embree Literary Services for her editorial skill, support, and unswerving enthusiasm during this effort. Robert Aulicino, who did the book cover design and layout, was indispensable. Their professional approach has made this effort easier than expected.

The text was translated into French by Laurence Petite of Boulder, Colorado. Ms. Petite's efforts were authoritative and professional in every respect.

Jonathan E. Jensen, MD FACP
Longmont, CO
September 24, 2004

TABLE OF CONTENTS

INTRODUCTION

If you listen to your patients, they will tell what is wrong. It is your job to understand what is being said and relate it to your knowledge.
—Wallace N. Jensen, MD MACP

Give me the uncle of your chicken!
—A tourist.

ALTHOUGH THE ABOVE QUOTES MAY SEEM COMPLETELY DISPARATE, THEY are actually quite closely related. The first quote is from my father, a Professor of Medicine and teacher of medicine for more than fifty years. He taught me the importance of listening to my patients and much more about the practice of medicine through the years.

The second quote is from a story related by a patient. It reflects misinterpretation of language despite the best of intentions. The story grew from his recent trip to Europe and the humorous events surrounding meals, transportation, and other challenges they faced in a foreign country. They did their best to speak the language but sometimes, obviously, came up a bit short.

With these two in mind, one can see the beauty, difficulty, and insight involved in any medical interview. The transfer of information between physician and patient constitutes a vital key in the practice of medicine. The selection of medical tests, interpretation of test results, and initiation of therapy are all based upon the initial medical interview.

This book is designed to assist patients in delivering pertinent medical information to a foreign healthcare provider. A medical interview between two persons who are speaking the same language can be confusing. The addition of a foreign language and social barrier will certainly further complicate this difficult situation.

While this book will help clarify communication between people who speak a different language, the patient should understand that no text can ever substitute for a complete medical history. If there is any doubt, an interpreter is always beneficial.

How to Use This Book

**Fill out as many sections of this book as you feel necessary.
Information is always useful to a physician.**

THE PURPOSE OF THIS BOOK IS TO ALLOW THE PATIENT, WHEN CHALLENGED with medical illness and a language barrier, to accurately explain his illness to a foreign physician. The medical information is based on the concepts of "pertinent positives and negatives." The format of the book is one of "yes" answers. By choosing only the "yes" answers, the "pertinent positives" (and hence "pertinent negatives") to a medical history are provided to the treating physician.

The book is structured in such a fashion as to provide this information without a two-way conversation in a foreign language. This text is not a substitute for a medical translator. The participants will be the only persons who can fully determine if adequate information has been exchanged.

It is my firm hope that you will not need this book during your travels. However, if you do it should provide you with the ability to rapidly communicate essential information to those providing healthcare.

Reviewing the guidelines prior to your departure will help provide important medical information to your physician. **Gathering and recording this information will assure that it is readily available when and if you need it during a medical emergency. You will not be able to collect this data while abroad. Now is the time to think about the guidelines and to obtain any other medical information that you think might be pertinent.**

Review all the sections of this book and become familiar with the layout and the contents. Be sure you understand how the text works and what it can (and cannot) do for you while traveling.

Two basic instructions (in addition to common sense) are carried out throughout this book. These are:

Check only those questions to which you answer "YES"

3

Circle all that apply

By reading through the text prior to completing a section and the above instructions you will maximize your transfer of information. The process may be tedious but it is important.

Have a safe and fulfilling trip.

TRAVEL GUIDELINES

What you need to do four to six weeks prior to departure

Arrange for an office visit with your physician
Inform the office of your travel needs prior to seeing the physician. This allows the medical office to make copies of any needed records and the physician the opportunity to dictate letters or provide any medical information which may be required for your travel. Office visits are the best method since they allow your physician to dedicate time needed to address your individual concerns and medical problems.

If you are traveling as a family, remember to contact your pediatrician or family practitioner regarding your children's medical conditions. A consultation with a travel medicine specialist for any vaccinations and recommendations is mandatory.

Further information about the prevention of medical problems can be obtained from several sources. The Center for Disease Control has up-to-date medical travel information. Their Web site is www.cdc.gov. The International Society for Travel Medicine (ISTM) has a list of members who specialize in Travel Medicine. Their website is www.ISTM.org. Click on the Travel Clinics (by location tab). This will allow access to a list of physican members by country. This reference is invaluable.

As we all know, medical illness is an unexpected event. Good outcomes are based upon anticipation and planning. Read this book and make all the preparations outlined, plus any of those you think are beneficial.

The following is the information you will need:
- Full name of your physician(s)
- Physician's address
- Physician's telephone and fax numbers and e-mail address
- Complete list of all current medications (brand and generic names), doses, and frequencies

5

- Your blood type
- A copy of your eyeglass prescription
- Complete list of all allergies—medical and environmental
- Complete list of all current and past medical problems. If you have a complicated medical problem, such as migraine headaches, write down the date, studies (CT scan, MRI, etc.) and pertinent results of these evaluations. Consider copying the reports to take with you on your trip.
- Complete list of any unusual medical events you have experienced.
- A letter from your physician, on his letterhead, listing any medications you will be taking with you during your travels
- List of all vaccinations and dates

Contact your insurance company
Request information regarding your insurance coverage while traveling abroad. What are the limitations of your policy? Can you get supplemental insurance to cover medical emergencies? Does your company have offices in your planned areas of travel? Obtain these phone numbers and record them in the appropriate sections within this book. Make three copies of all of the above information.

Leave one copy with someone in the United States who will be available to assist you should it be necessary. This person should also have a copy of all your passports, visas, itinerary, emergency contacts, credit cards, etc. In the event that you become incapacitated and require such assistance, this information is extremely valuable. You might wish to discuss such a situation with a lawyer prior to departure.

The second copy should be with your extra copy of all your passports, visas, emergency contacts, etc. If loss of one copy occurs, you are assured of adequate information regarding your credit cards, passports, and other important documents.

Place the third copy with *Globetrotter's Pocket Doc*.

DEALING WITH MEDICAL PROBLEMS WHILE ABROAD

BOTH MAJOR AND MINOR MEDICAL PROBLEMS OCCUR FREQUENTLY. Furthermore, you may need to make medical decisions regarding your health and/or those of your traveling companions. In all situations, consider whether this can be treated without a physician (such as replacement of lost medications, requesting cold remedies, etc.) or by a physician (chest pain, abdominal pain, etc.). After this decision has been made, select the appropriate section of this book for further assistance.

To effectively get help abroad, you must be able to communicate. Paramount to this is written pertinent information about your personal health. **Please do not neglect to fill out the sections on medical history**. If you have no known allergies to medications, write in the allergy section "No Known Drug Allergies (NKDA)." If the section is left blank, a physician may not know whether it has not yet been filled out or is truly negative. **Complete all of these forms!**

If you are traveling with a family, copy the forms you will be using from this book and fill them out for each family member.

When obtaining any medical care, follow these guidelines.
- Introduce yourself using the Patient Introduction Section.
- Allow the healthcare provider to read the Physician Introduction. This section introduces the text and how it may provide assistance.
- Be sure to show the Medical History Section to the healthcare provider.
- Select the section(s) most appropriate to your complaints.
- Read through the section first to be sure that you have selected correctly.
- Read through a second time, checking the appropriate boxes only for YES answers.
- Circle any multiple choice sections within a question. Follow the rule, "Circle all that apply." This format is kept throughout the book and allows for pertinent "positives" and "negatives" to

be translated to the provider.
- Be polite and patient. You are in a difficult situation that may try your patience and cause anxiety. Being rude does not help.

Minor Medical Problems

Minor medical problems occur frequently. If a child has a runny nose or a cold, formal medical consultation may not be required. Many parents are well educated in the diagnosis and treatment of their children's minor health problems. A simple trip to the local pharmacy may be all that is required to solve the problem.

Unfortunately, the pharmacy in a foreign country is not the typical pharmacy in the United States. Although a parent may know that Robutussin works quite well for their child's cold, Robitussin may not be available in another country. Many medications are similar. The differences may include dose, frequency, name and combination of drugs within a specific preparation. However, finding the appropriate medication requires communication with the pharmacist. This text has a comprehensive list of over-the-counter medications, generic names, and the translation. Every effort has been made to ensure that these are accurate.

As an example, let us assume that Billy, your 16-year-old son, has a common cold successfully managed in the USA with Aleve Cold and Sinus medicine. In this case, you can use the Personal Information Section to describe to the pharmacist the age, sex, weight, and familial relation of the child. Next, you would proceed to the Minor Complaint Section and report to the pharmacist that he has a cold. A quick look in the Non-Prescription Medication Section will show a variety of medications that are used to treat this condition, including the preferred Aleve Cold and Sinus. By showing the pharmacist this information, an appropriate substitute can be identified. What is the end result? A grateful son, a happy family, and a vacation that continues on as planned.

Always use the Personal Medical History Section of this book when discussing any health related matter while in a foreign country. **It is advisable to fill this out for all travelers prior to leaving the country. This ensures that the data is available to anyone who might need it quickly.**

Major Medical Problems

Globetrotter's Pocket Doc assists with these needs by providing descriptions of acute medical problem, personal medical history information, and a prescription medication translation section. The questions may seem tedious. However, by answering all these questions, the physician will be able to ascertain important information, not only from the "Yes" answers (those that have been checked or circled) but also by the negatives (the ones that have not been checked or circled.) This is a basic technique used during the medical interview. It allows a physician to understand what is called "the pertinent positives and negatives" of a medical history. In addition, the prescription medication section contains about 200 commonly prescribed medications, their generic names, and translations. Every effort has been made to ensure the accuracy of these medications and their translations.

IMPORTANT BASIC INFORMATION FORMS

Health Insurance

Name of Insurance Carrier _____

Home office street address _____

City_____State _____

Country _____ Zip code _____

Phone number _____

Fax number _____

Email address _____

Policy number _____ Group number_____

Group insured (company) _____

Local office street address _____

City _____ State _____

Country _____ Zip code _____

Phone number _____

Fax number _____

Email address _____

Policy number_____ Group number_____

Group insured (company) _____

Personal Information

Name _____

Title _____

Date of birth _____

Street address _____

City _____ State _____

Country _____ Zip code _____

Home phone number _____

Fax number _____

Email address _____

I am traveling on (check one)

❏ business   ❏ pleasure

I am traveling with (check one)

❏ friends   ❏ my family   ❏ business associates   ❏ alone

Business name _____

Business street address _____

City _____ State _____

Country _____ Zip Code_____

Business contact _____

Telephone _____

Fax number _____

Email address _____

Local Information

Name of hotel or temporary residence _____

Street address _____

City_____ State _____

Country_____ Zip Code _____

Telephone _____

Fax number_____

Email address _____

Emergency Contact Information (Local)

Name_____

Street address _____

City _____ State _____

Country _____ Zip Code _____

Telephone _____

Fax number _____

Email address _____

Business _____

Business Telephone _____

Emergency Contact Information (United States)

Name _____

Street address _____

City _____ State _____

Country _____ Zip Code_____

Telephone _____

Fax number _____

Email address _____

Business _____

Business Telephone_____

Other Relatives or Contacts

Name_____Relationship _____

Street address _____

City _____ State _____

Country_____Zip Code _____

Home phone number _____

Fax number _____

Email address _____

Business phone number _____

Fax number _____

Email address _____

Personal Medical Information

Personal Physician _____

Specialty _____

Street address _____

City _____ State _____

Country _____ Zip Code _____

Phone number _____

Fax number _____

Email address _____

Consulting Physician _____

Specialty _____

Street address _____

City _____ State _____

Country _____ Zip Code _____

Phone number _____

Fax number _____

Email address _____

Medical History

Event   Date

_____

_____

_____

_____

_____

_____

Surgical History

Event   Date

_____

_____

_____

_____

_____

_____

Hospitalizations

Reason for Admission   Date

_____

_____

_____

_____

_____

_____

Medications

Medication   Dose   Frequency

_____

_____

_____

_____

_____

_____

Allergies

Medication   Type of Reaction to Medication

_____

_____

_____

_____

_____

Vaccinations

Vaccination   Date

_____

_____

_____

_____

_____

_____

Immunizations
(especially important for children)

Immunization   Date

_____

_____

_____

_____

_____

_____

PHYSICIAN INTRODUCTION

Dear Physician,

Having been in exactly the position you are presently in, I have written this book to assist those traveling in foreign countries in furnishing their medical information. It is designed to provide some basic information regarding medical problems which are likely to cause a patient to request professional assistance.

The book is designed to provide a good medical history, "pertinent positives" and, by elimination, "pertinent negatives." In the front of the book, the patient should have completed information forms regarding their medical history, medications, allergies, etc. There is no family history form included since most acute medical problems will not require this information.

This book is not a comprehensive review of the history. Hopefully, it will provide you with enough information to make an accurate diagnosis without a translator. However, only you can make a decision regarding the need for such services during a medical evaluation.

Since many patients will require follow-up care upon returning home, this text will also serve as a guide for their hometown physician.

I hope that this text is helpful to you.

Sincerely,

Jonathan E. Jensen, MD FACP
Board Certified Internal Medicine
Board Certified Gastroenterology
Clinical Associate Professor of Medicine
    University Health Sciences Center of Colorado
    Denver, Colorado

PRÉSENTATION DU MÉDECIN

Cher/ère collègue,

Pour m'être trouvé dans la même situation que celle dans laquelle vous vous trouvez en ce moment, j'ai écrit cet ouvrage pour aider les patients voyageant à l'étranger à fournir des renseignements sur leur état de santé. Cet ouvrage a été conçu pour fournir des renseignements de base concernant des problèmes médicaux susceptibles de nécessiter une assistance médicale.

Ce livre a été conçu pour faire apparaître clairement les antécédents médicaux du patient ainsi que les symptômes importants et, par élimination, l'absence de symptômes importants. Au début du livre, le patient devra avoir rempli un questionnaire médical indiquant ses antécédents médicaux, ses traitements en cours, ses allergies, etc. Cet ouvrage n'inclut pas les antécédents familiaux car la plupart des problèmes médicaux sérieux ne nécessitent pas ce genre de renseignements.

Ce livre ne prétend pas donner une liste exhaustive de tous les antécédents médicaux. Mais il vous fournira, je l'espère, suffisamment de renseignements pour vous permettre de faire un diagnostic correct sans avoir besoin d'un traducteur. Il va de soi, néanmoins, que vous seul êtes à même de prendre une décision concernant la nécessité d'avoir recours aux services d'un traducteur durant le bilan médical.

Etant donné que de nombreux patients nécessiteront un suivi médical à leur retour aux Etats-Unis, cet ouvrage servira également de guide à leur médecin de famille lorsqu'ils rentreront.

En espérant que cet ouvrage vous sera utile.

Sincères salutations,

Jonathan E. Jensen, Docteur en Médecine
(FACP: Fellow of the American College of Physicians)
Diplômé en Médecine Interne
Diplômé en Gastro-entérologie

PATIENT INTRODUCTION
(For minor medical problems)

This section is designed to provide a basic introduction to a health-care professional, such as a pharmacist. Use this section when obtaining information and medical assistance for minor medical problems. If you use this section for major medical problems, it is advisable to review all the chapters of the book and to complete those which appear appropriate.

Always complete the sections on your medical history, medications, and allergies. This is vital information for any medical consultation whether it is minor or major in nature.

SECTION CONCERNANT VOTRE ENTRÉE EN MATIÈRE
(pour des problèmes médicaux mineurs)

Cette section a pour but de vous aider à vous présenter sommairement au professionnel de la santé. Cette section est très utile pour des problèmes médicaux mineurs nécessitant, par exemple, une visite à la pharmacie. Utilisez cette section pour obtenir des informations ainsi qu'une assistance médicale pour des problèmes médicaux mineurs. Vous pouvez aussi utiliser cette section pour des problèmes médicaux majeurs. Si vous utilisez cette section pour des problèmes médicaux majeurs, il vous est conseillé de passer en revue tous les chapitres de ce livre et de compléter ceux qui semblent vous concerner.

Veillez à toujours compléter les sections concernant vos antécédents médicaux, vos traitements en cours, et vos allergies, etc. Ces renseignements sont d'une importance capitale pour toute consultation médicale, quel que soit le degré de gravité du problème.

Hello, my name is: _____

Bonjour, je m'appelle: _____

Would you be kind enough to assist me? I do not speak your
language.

Voulez-vous avoir la gentillesse de m'aider, s'il vous plait? Je ne
parle pas votre langue.

Please read through the Physicians Introduction. This will help us
understand each other.

Auriez-vous l'amabilité de lire l'introduction du médecin? Cela
facilitera la communication.

I am here on behalf of:

Je viens vous consulter pour:

❏ myself.
  moi-même.
❏ my son/daughter.
  mon fils/ma fille.
❏ my husband/wife.
  mon mari/ma femme.
❏ my friend.
  mon ami(e).

The patient is _____ years of age.

Le patient a _____ ans.

The patient weighs _____ lb/kg. (2.2 pounds = 1 kilogram)

Le patient pèse _____ lb/kg.

The patient has: (check all that apply)

Le patient a: (cochez tout ce qui convient)

❏ a cold.
  le rhume.
❏ a runny nose.
  le nez qui coule.
❏ sinusitis.
  sinusite.
❏ a headache.
  mal à la tête.
❏ a sore throat.

mal à la gorge.
❏ an earache.
mal aux oreilles.
❏ scratchy eyes
les yeux qui piquent.
❏ chills.
des frissons.
❏ sweats.
des suées.
❏ a cough.
une toux.
❏ vomiting.
des vomissements.
❏ diarrhea.
la diarrhée.
❏ fever.
de la fièvre.
❏ heartburn.
des brûlures d'estomac.
❏ allergies.
des allergies.
❏ aches and pains in the muscles and joints.
des courbatures et des douleurs dans les muscles et les
articulations.
❏ dehydration.
une déshydratation.

Choose one of the following options:

1. In the United States, the patient would take this medication. (Turn to the appropriate page in the Non-Prescription or Prescription Medication Section.) Can you find something that would be similar or might work for this problem? I appreciate your help and patience. Thank you very much.

1. Aux Etats-Unis, le patient prendrait ce médicament. (Aller à la page correspondante dans la section concernant les médicaments délivrés sur ordonnance ou en vente libre). Pourriez-vous lui prescrire un médicament semblable, ou quelque chose qui résoudrait le problème? Merci beaucoup de prendre le temps de m'aider ainsi.

2. I am not sure what medication I would use in the United States. Could you please assist me with selecting a medication that would be of benefit? I appreciate your help and patience. Thank you very much.

2. Je ne sais pas quel médicament j'utiliserais aux Etats-Unis. Pourriez-vous m'aider à trouver un médicament qui soulagerait le partient? Merci beaucoup de prendre le temps de m'aider ainsi.

LOST MEDICATIONS

The following section is supplied for individuals who have lost their medications. Complete the above introductory section. Also, be sure that you have completed all of the sections in the front to the best of your ability. This type of information is very valuable to healthcare professionals.

A limited prescription medications list (with translations) is available in the back of the book. If possible, bring a letter from your personal physician that can confirm the need for these medications.

Be patient. Ensuring that the right medications are provided may take some time. Not all medications available in the United States are available in other countries.

AU CAS OÙ VOUS PERDRIEZ VOS MÉDICAMENTS

La section suivante concerne les personnes qui ont perdu leurs médicaments. Complétez la section ci-dessus concernant votre entrée en matière. Assurez-vous également d'avoir complété avec le plus grand soin les sections figurant en début de livre. Ce type de renseignements est très important pour les professionnels de la santé.

Une petite liste de médicaments delivrés sur ordonnance (avec leur traduction) figure en fin de livre. Si possible, apportez une lettre de votre médecin personnel confirmant la nécessité pour vous de prendre ces médicaments.

Soyez patient(e). Le fait de vérifier que l'on vous prescrit bien les médicaments qui s'imposent peut prendre du temps. Les médicaments disponibles aux Etats-Unis ne sont pas forcément tous disponibles dans les autres pays.

Hello, my name is _____

Bonjour, je m'appelle _____

Would you be kind enough to assist me? I do not speak your
   language.

Voulez-vous avoir la gentillesse de m'aider, s'il vous plait?
   Je ne parle pas votre langue.

Please read the Physicians Introduction. This will help us understand
   each other.

Auriez-vous l'amabilité de lire l'introduction du médecin? Cela facilitera la communication.

I am here on behalf of:

Je viens vous consulter pour:

- ❏ myself.
  moi-même.
- ❏ my son/daughter.
  mon fils/ma fille.
- ❏ my husband/wife.
  mon mari/ma femme.
- ❏ my friend.
  mon ami(e).

The patient is _____ years of age.

Le patient a _____ ans.

The patient weighs _____ lb/kg. (2.2 pounds = 1 kilogram)

Le patient pèse _____ lb/kg.

- ❏ The patient has lost his/her medications. Would you please help me in replacing them? I appreciate your help and patience with this matter. Thank you very much.
  Le patient a perdu ses médicaments. Pourriez-vous, s'il vous plaît, m'aider à remplacer ces médicaments? Merci beaucoup de prendre le temps de m'aider ainsi.
- ❏ The patient takes these medications. (Show the medication list to the healthcare professional.)
  Le patient prend ces médicaments-ci. (Montrer la liste des médicaments au professionnel de la santé.)
- ❏ Could you please sell me enough medications to last for the next _____ days?
  Pourriez-vous, s'il vous plaît, me vendre suffisamment de médicaments pour les _____ prochains jours?
- ❏ If you cannot provide me with these medications, would you please write down the address of a physician or hospital where I can get the prescriptions filled?
  Si vous ne pouvez pas me fournir ces médicaments, pourriez-vous, s'il vous plaît, m'indiquer l'adresse d'un médecin ou d'un hôpital où je pourrais obtenir une ordonnance?

❏ Thank you very much for your kind assistance. I am very grateful for your patience and help.

Merci de votre aide. Je vous suis très reconnaissant(e) de m'aider ainsi.

CHARTS, SCALES AND DIAGRAMS

Visual Field Diagram

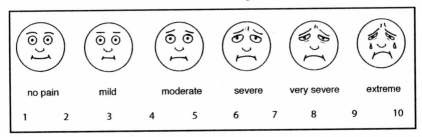

Temperature Scale

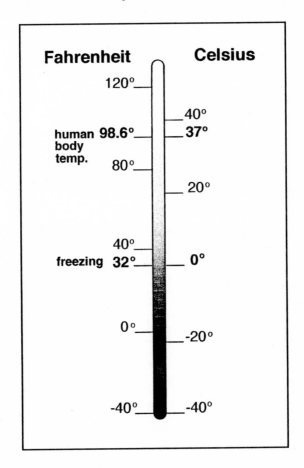

Metric Conversion Chart

when you know	multiply by	to find
	LENGTH	
inches	2.5	centimeters
feet	30	centimeters
yards	0.9	meters
miles	1.6	kilometers
centimeters	0,393	inches
meters	1.1	yards
kilometers	0.6	miles
	WEIGHT	
ounces	28	grams
pounds	0.45	kilograms
grams	0.035	ounces
kilograms	2.2	pounds
	VOLUME	
teaspoons	5	milliliters
tablespoons	15	milliliters
fluid ounces	30	milliliters
cups	0.24	liters
pints	0.47	liters
quarts	0.95	liters
gallons	3.8	liters
milliliters	0.034	fluid ounce
liters	2.1	pints, US
liters	1.76	pints, Imp.
liters	1.06	quarts,US
liters	0.88	quarts,Imp.
liters	0.26	gallons,US
liters	0.22	gallons,Imp.

Imp.-Imperial System
US -USA System

Visual Pain Scale

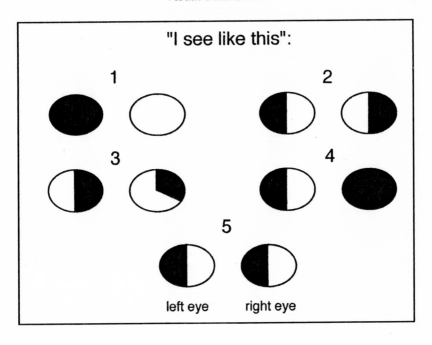

ANATOMIC DIAGRAMS

Head Diagrams

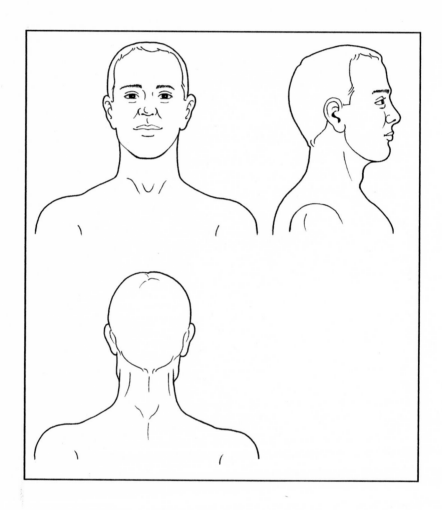

Face Diagram

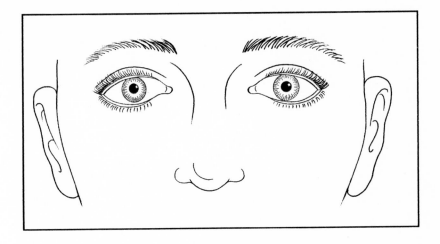

Neck Diagrams

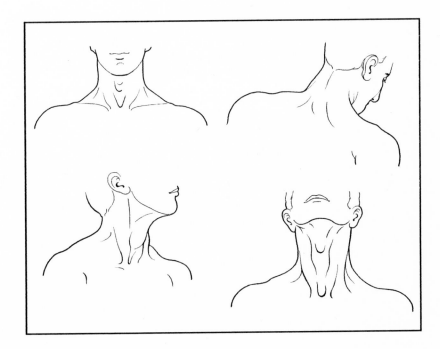

Chest and Back Diagrams

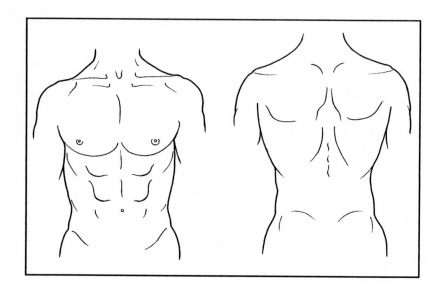

Abdominal Diagram

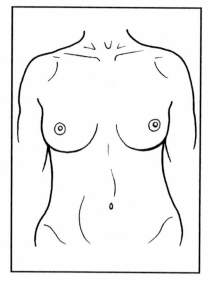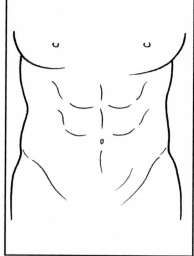

Groin Diagrams

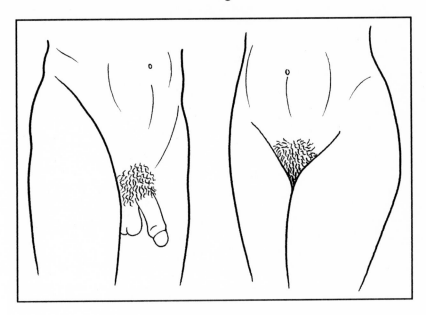

Shoulder Diagrams

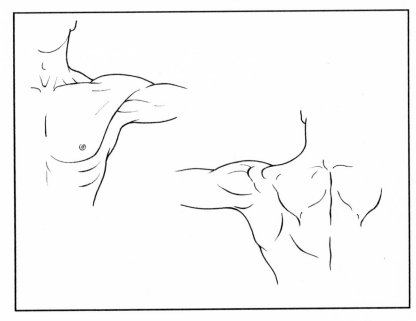

Arm Diagrams

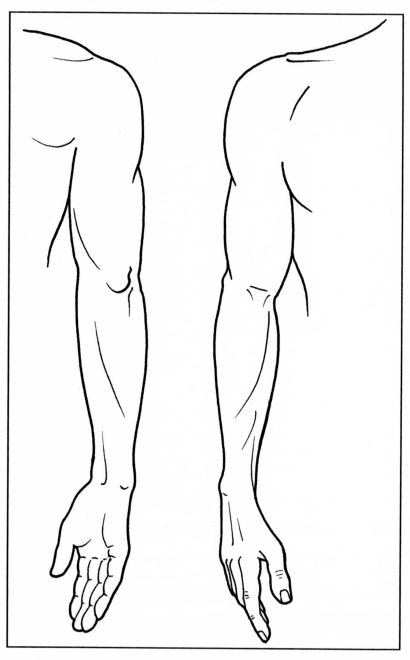

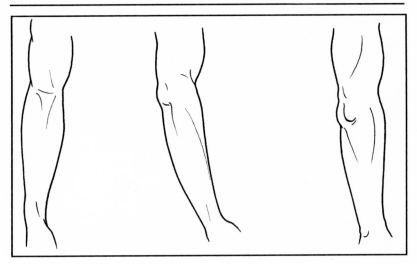

Hand Diagrams

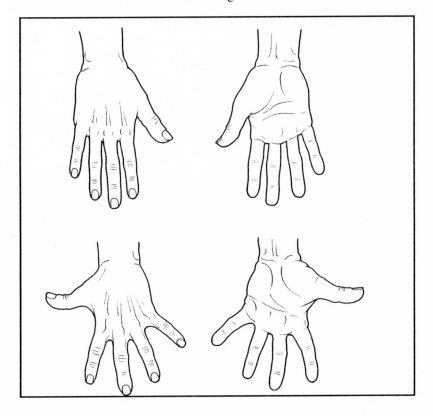

Leg Diagrams

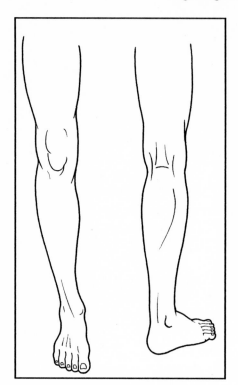

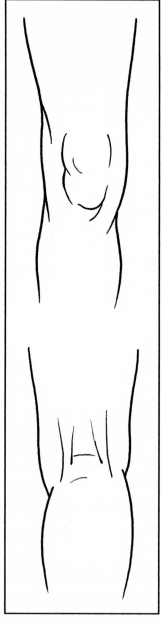

Foot Diagrams

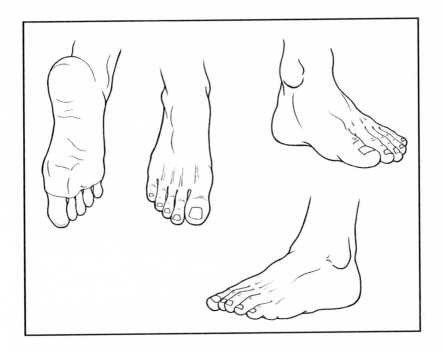

MAJOR PEDIATRIC COMPLAINTS

Please be sure that the forms regarding your child's medical history, current medications, allergies, etc. have been filled out completely. The information in this section is invaluable to all health care providers. The more information you provide the better the decision. If you feel that it might benefit your health, answer more than one section.

Pediatric Fever

A fever in a child is usually a sign that there is an infection somewhere. Teething can also be a cause of fever. The fever itself is not a problem or a danger to the child. The infection causing the fever may or may not be a serious problem. It is more important to look for the cause of the fever than to treat it. The fever does not cause brain damage as is commonly believed. Treating the fever may make a child feel better but will not improve the underlying problem. A fever that will not "break" with medications does not signify a more serious disease. Fevers in children under three months of age can be particularly serious because of their immature immune system.

Acetaminophen or ibuprofen may be used for comfort. These are available in most countries without a prescription. You should have these in a medical kit for travel. Do not use cool baths or alcohol to cool a child.

Les fièvres infantiles

La fièvre chez l'enfant est généralement le signe qu'il y a une infection quelque part. Un enfant qui fait ses dents peut aussi avoir de la fièvre. Le fièvre en elle-même n'est ni problématique, ni dangereuse. En revanche, l'infection qui est la cause de la fièvre peut, dans certains cas, être grave. Il est plus important de déterminer la cause de la fièvre que de la traiter. La fièvre n'entraîne pas de dommages au cervau comme on le croit vulgairement. Le traitement de la fièvre peut en effet soulager l'enfant, mais le problème de fond n'a pas été réglé. Une fièvre qui ne "s'arrête" pas sous l'effet des médicaments n'est pas le signe d'une maladie plus grave. Les fièvres chez les enfants de moins de trois mois peuvent être particulièrement graves en raison de leur système immunitaire immature.

On peut donner à l'enfant de l'acétaminophène ou de l'ibuprofène pour le soulager. On peut se procurer ces médicaments sans ordonnance dans la plupart des pays. Veillez à en avoir dans votre trousse à médicaments pour le voyage. Ne pas faire prendre à l'enfant de bains d'eau fraîche, ni ne le frictionner avec de l'alcool pour le rafraîchir.

Check only those questions to which you answer YES.
Cochez seulement les questions auxquelles vous répondez OUI.

Complaint
Symptômes
Child's age: _____
  (months or years)
Age de l'enfant: _____
  (mois ou ans)
My child has a fever of _____.
  (Refer to Temperature Scale)
Mon enfant a de la fièvre _____.
  (Voir l'échelle de temperature)
He/she has had fever
  for _____ minutes/hours/days.
Il/elle a de la fièvre depui
  _____ minutes/heures/jours.

I have given the following
  medications:
❏ Acetaminophen
❏ Ibuprofen
❏ Other _____
Je lui ai donné ces
  médicaments-ci:
  Acétaminophène
  Ibuprofène
  Autres _____

Other symptoms

Autres symptômes

❑ Crying

Mon enfant pleure.

❑ Drooling

Mon enfant bave

❑ Teething

Mon enfant fait ses dents.

❑ Runny nose

Mon enfant a le nez qui coule.

❑ Cough

Mon enfant tousse.

❑ Rash

Mon enfant a de l'urticaire.

❑ Vomiting

Mon enfant vomit.

❑ Child has been vomiting for ___ hours.

Mon enfant vomit depuis ___ heures.

❑ Child has vomited___ times.

Mon enfant a vomi ___ fois.

❑ Diarrhea

Mon enfant a la diarrhée.

❑ Child has had diarrhea for ___ hours.

Mon enfant a la diarrhée depuis ___ heures.

❑ Child has had ___ stools (dirty diapers) today.

Mon enfant a fait ___ selles (a fait dans sa couche fois) aujourd'hui.

Feeding

Alimentation

❑ Child will eat or drink normally.

Mon enfant boit et mange normalement.

❑ Child will drink but not eat.

Mon enfant boit mais ne mange pas.

❑ Child does not eat or drink well.

Mon enfant ne mange et ne boit pas beaucoup.

❏ Child does not eat or drink at all.

Mon enfant ne mange et ne boit pas du tout.

Pediatric Vomiting/Diarrhea

Vomiting and diarrhea are very common in children. They are most often the result of an infection (gastroenteritis). This can be caused by a virus or bacteria. Bacteria are a common cause of "travelers diarrhea." These infections can be caught from other people or from food or water. "Food poisoning" is a form of gastroenteritis. Vomiting can be from other causes such as an intestinal blockage, intestinal bleeding, or appendicitis.

The main concern with treating gastroenteritis is keeping the child hydrated. The American Academy of Pediatrics recommends continuing fluids even if the child is still vomiting. Small frequent amounts of fluids work best. When the child is able to tolerate fluids well, you should try to advance to regular foods. You should encourage feeding even if the diarrhea continues. Milk or formula had traditionally been avoided in the past. However, there is little evidence that it is bad, and it is often the only liquid a child will take. Intravenous hydration in the hospital is sometimes required. This is common in the United States and is probably overused. It is rarely done in other countries where oral hydration is preferred.

Medications are not commonly used for these conditions. The problem should be self resolving.

Les vomissements/diarrhées infantiles

Les vomissements et les diarrhées sont très courants chez l'enfant. Ils sont le plus souvent la conséquence d'une infection (gastro-entérite), qui peut être virale ou bactérielle. Les bactéries sont une cause fréquente de la "diarrhée du voyageur." Ces infections peuvent s'attraper au contact d'autres personnes ou par de la nourriture ou de l'eau. "L'empoisonnement alimentaire" est une forme de gastro-entérite. Les vomissements peuvent être dus à d'autres causes comme une occlusion intestinale, un saignement intestinal ou une appendicite.

Pour traiter une gastro-entérite, le plus important est de veiller à ce que l'enfant reste hydraté. La Société Américaine de Pédiatrie recommande de continuer à donner des fluides à l'enfant même s'il vomit encore. Le mieux est de lui donner fréquemment de petites quantités de fluides. Quand l'enfant est en mesure de bien tolérer les fluides, passez alors à de la nourriture normale. Il faut encourager l'enfant à s'alimenter même si la diarrhée continue. Traditionnellement, on évitait le lait et le lait maternisé, mais il n'est pas prouvé que cela soit mauvais et c'est souvent le seul liquide que l'enfant accepte de boire. Il faut parfois avoir recours à une hydratation par intra-veineuse à l'hôpital. Cela se pratique fréquemment aux Etats-Unis, et l'on a probablement recours à cette solution trop souvent. Cela n'est pas très fréquent dans d'autres pays où l'on préfère l'hydratation par voie orale.

On n'utilise généralement pas de médicaments pour ce genre de problème qui, normalement, finit par se résoudre tout seul.

Check only those questions to which you answer YES.
Cochez seulement les questions auxquelles vous répondez OUI.

Complaint
Symptômes
Child's age____(months or years)
   Age de l'enfant: ____ (mois ou ans)
Child's normal weight: ____
   Poids normal de l'enfant: ____
❑ My child is vomiting. It has been going on for_____
   minutes/hours/days.
   Mon enfant vomit. Cela dure depuis____ minutes/heures/jours.
   Child has vomited ____ times.
   Mon enfant a vomi ____ fois.
❑ My child has diarrhea. It has been going on for____ min/hrs/days.
   There are ____ loose stools in one day.
   Mon enfant a la diarrhée.Cela dure depuis_____
   minutes/heures/jours.
   Il/elle a fait ____ selles molles en une journée.
❑ My child has abdominal pain. It has been going on for_____
   minutes/hours/days. (Refer to Visual Pain Scale)
   Mon enfant a des douleurs abdominales.
   Cela dure depuis ____(minutes/heures/jours) (Voir l'échelle de

douleur.)

The pain is

La douleur est

❏ constant

    constante

❏ intermittent

    intermittente

❏ My child has a fever (Refer to Temperature Scale)

    Mon enfant a de la fièvre (Voir l'échelle de temperature)

❏ My child will not take any fluids.

    Mon enfant ne supporte pas les fluids.

❏ My child will take fluids well.

    Mon enfant supporte bien les fluids.

I have been giving:

Je lui ai donné:

❏ water

    de l'eau

❏ formula

    du lait maternisé

❏ milk

    du lait

❏ juice

    du jus de fruit

❏ other: _____

    autre chose: _____

❏ My child will eat.

    Mon enfant mange normalement.

❏ My child will not eat.

    Mon enfant ne mange pas.

❏ My child last urinated ____hours ago.

    Mon enfant a uriné pour la dernière fois il y a ____ heures.

I have given the following medications:

Je lui ai donné des medicaments:

❏ Acetaminophen

    Acétaminophène

❏ Ibuprofen
  Ibuprofène
❏ Pepto-bismol
  Pepto-bismol

Seizures in the Child

Seizures in the child are usually benign. Nevertheless, a complete evaluation is usually warranted. Many pediatric seizures are related to temperature (febrile seizures). See the section on Seizures in the Adult. Fill out the weight, age, and temperature. Please be sure that the first section regarding your medical history, current medications, allergies, etc. has been filled out completely.

Les attaques cérébrales chez l'enfant

Les attaques cérébrales chez l'enfant sont généralement bénignes. Néanmoins, un examen complet se justifie le plus souvent. De nombreuses attaques cérébrales infantiles sont liées à la température (attaques cérébrales fébriles). Consulter la section concernant les attaques cérébrales dans la section concernant les adultes. Indiquez le poids et l'âge. Veuillez vous assurer d'avoir complété soigneusement la première section concernant vos antécédents médicaux, vos traitements en cours, et vos allergies, etc. Les renseignements contenus dans cette section sont d'une importance capitale pour tout praticien de la santé.

Pediatric Cough/Difficulty Breathing

A cough in a child is usually a sign that there is a respiratory infection. Other causes may be asthma (if the child has a history of this) or choking. Most respiratory infections are caused by viruses and cannot be treated with antibiotics. Fortunately, these are not usually serious. Upper respiratory infections cause runny nose, cough, sore throat, and ear pain. There may be fever. Respiratory infections can become serious if they cause difficulty with breathing. Pneumonia is an infection in the lungs. This can be caused by viruses or bacteria and may need to be treated with antibiotics.

Les toux/problèmes respiratoires infantiles

La toux chez l'enfant est généralement le signe qu'il y a une infection respiratoire. La toux peut aussi être causée par de l'asthme (si l'enfant est asthmatique), ou par une suffocation. La plupart des infections respiratoires sont causées par des virus et ne peuvent pas être traitées par des antibiotiques. Heureusement, elles ne sont généralement pas graves. Les infections respiratoires supérieures se caractérisent pas le nez qui coule, une toux, des maux de gorge, et des douleurs dans les oreilles en plus de la toux. Elles peuvent s'accompagner de fièvre. Les infections respiratoires peuvent devenir graves si elles entraînent des problèmes respiratoires. La pneumonie est une infection des poumons. Elle peut être causée par des virus ou des bactéries et peut parfois nécessiter un traitement antibiotique.

Check only those questions to which you answer YES.
Cochez seulement les questions auxquelles vous répondez OUI.

Complaint
Symptômes
Child's age:____(months or years)
   Age de l'enfant:____(Mois ou ans)
❏ My child has a cough.
   It has been going on for ____ minutes/hours/days.
   Mon enfant tousse. Il/elle tousse depuis ____min/heures/jours.
❏ My child has difficulty breathing.
   Mon enfant a du mal à respirer.
❏ The cough is worse at night.
   Il/elle tousse le plus pendant la nuit.
❏ The cough is worse during the day.
   Il/elle tousse le plus pendant la journée.
I have given these medications:
   ❏ Acetaminophen
   ❏ Ibuprofen
   ❏ Other: _____
   Je lui ai donné ces médicaments-ci:
    Acétaminophène
    Ibuprofène
    Autres: _____

Other symptoms:
- ❏ Crying
- ❏ Drooling
- ❏ Teething
- ❏ Runny nose

Autres symptômes:
      Mon enfant pleure
      Mon enfant bave
      Mon enfant fait ses dents
      Mon enfant a le nez qui coule

❏ My child has a fever.
    (Refer to Temperature Scale)
  Mon enfant a de la fièvre.
    (Voir l'échelle de temperature)

❏ My child has a rash.
  Mon enfant a de l'urticaire.

❏ My child has a headache.
  Mon enfant a mal à la tête.

❏ My child has an earache.
  Mon enfant a mal aux oreilles.

❏ My child has been vomiting.
    Mon enfant vomit.
  My child has been vomiting for ____ hours.
    Mon enfant vomit depuis____ heures.
  The child has vomited____ times.
    Mon enfant a vomi ____ fois.

Pediatric Abdominal Pain

Abdominal pain in a child is common and is usually not a serious problem. There are several serious causes of abdominal pain. Appendicitis causes pain in the right lower part of the abdomen and is usually associated with fever. Appendicitis needs to be treated with surgery. An intestinal blockage can occur in very young children. There is pain, vomiting, and either no diarrhea or blood in the diarrhea. Intestinal infections can cause pain as well as vomiting and lots of diarrhea.

Les douleurs abdominales infantiles

Les douleurs abdominales chez l'enfant sont fréquentes et ne sont généralement pas graves. Il y a toutefois plusieurs causes graves de douleurs abdominales. L'appendicite provoque une douleur dans la partie inférieure droite de l'abdomen qui s'accompagne généralement de fièvre. Une appendicite nécessite d'être traitée par une opération. Une occlusion intestinale peut survenir chez les très jeunes enfants. On constate alors des douleurs, des vomissements, l'absence de diarrhées ou, au contraire, des diarrhées sanglantes. Les infections intestinales peuvent provoquer des douleurs, des vomissements et des diarrhées abondantes.

Check only those questions to which you answer YES.
Cochez seulement les questions auxquelles vous répondez OUI.

Complaint
Symptômes
Child's age:____(months or years)
Age de l'enfant:____(Mois ou ans)
❏ My child has abdominal pain.
It has been going on for ____minutes/hours/days.
  (Refer to Visual Pain Scale)
  Mon enfant a des douleurs abdominales.
  Il/elle a mal depuis ____ min/heures/jours.
  (Voir echelle de douleur)
❏ The pain is constant.
  La douleur est constante.
❏ The pain comes and goes.
  La douleur va et vient.
The pain is:
  ❏ sharp
  ❏ dull
  ❏ burning
La douleur est:
  aiguë
  sourde
  cuisante

❑ The pain is everywhere.

Il/elle a mal partout.

The pain is located _____

(Refer to Abdominal Diagram)

La douleur se situe ____

(Voir la diagramme de l'abdomen)

❑ My child has had this pain before (give dates) _____

Mon enfant a déjà eu mal comme cela (préciser les dates)_____

❑ My child has had abdominal surgery.

Mon enfant a déjà subi une opération de l'abdomen.

❑ My child has had an appendectomy.

Mon enfant a déjà subi une opération de l'appendicite (appendicectomie).

❑ My child has a fever.

(Refer to Temperature Scale)

Mon enfant a de la fièvre.

(Voir l'échelle de temperature)

My child has been vomiting for____ hours.

Mon enfant vomit depuis____ heures.

My child has vomited____times.

Mon enfant a vomi____ fois.

❑ My child has diarrhea. (Refer to Pediatric Vomiting/Diarrhea Section)

Mon enfant a la diarrhea.(Voir les vomissements/diarrhées infantiles)

❑ My child has been crying.

Mon enfant pleure.

❑ My child has been drooling.

Mon enfant bave.

❑ My child is teething.

Mon enfant fait ses dents.

❑ My child has a runny nose.

Mon enfant a le nez qui coule.

❑ My child has a rash.

Mon enfant a de l'urticaire.

❏ My child has a headache.
   Mon enfant a mal à la tête.
❏ My child has an earache.
   Mon enfant a mal aux oreilles.
I have given the following
   medications:
   ❏ Acetaminophen
   ❏ Ibuprofen
   ❏ Other: _____
      Je lui ai donné ces médicaments-ci:
         Acétaminophène
         Ibuprofène
         Autres: _____

GENERAL COMPLAINTS: ADULT

Introduction
This section reviews general problems that commonly accompany other medical problems. This section, which covers dehydration, fever, nausea, and vomiting, will be referred to in many areas of the book.

Please be sure that the first section regarding your medical history, current medications, allergies, etc. has been filled out completely. The information contained within this section is invaluable to all health care providers. The more information you provide, the better the decision. If you feel it might benefit your health, answer more than one section.

PROBLÈMES GÉNÉRAUX: ADULTE

Introduction
Cette section passe en revue les problèmes généraux qui accompagnent souvent d'autres problèmes médicaux. De nombreuses parties de ce livre feront référence à cette section. Cette section couvre la déshydration, la fièvre, les nausées et les vomissements.

Veuillez vous assurer d'avoir complété soigneusement la section I concernant vos antécédents médicaux, vos traitements en cours, et vos allergies, etc. Les renseignements contenus dans cette section sont d'une importance capitale pour tout praticien de la santé. Plus les renseignements fournis seront nombreux, meilleure sera la décision prise par le praticien. Si vous pensez que cela peut être dans l'intérêt de votre santé, ne vous limitez pas à une section, complétez-en plusieurs.

Dehydration
Dehydration is a common problem which may occur alone or secondary to other medical conditions such as infectious diarrhea.

La déshydratation
La déshydratation est un problème courant pouvant survenir seul ou à la suite d'autres problèmes de santé tels que les diarrhées infectieuses.

Check only those questions to which you answer YES.
Cochez seulement les questions auxquelles vous répondez OUI.

Complaint
Symptômes
❏ I am dehydrated.
   Je suis déshydraté(e).

Associated symptoms and history:
Symptômes associés et information complémentaires:
❏ My face is flushed.
   J'ai des rougeurs au visage.
❏ I have been very thirsty.
   J'ai très soif.
❏ I have been urinating frequently.
   J'urine fréquemment.
❏ My urine is very dark.
   Mon urine est très sombre.
❏ I feel weak.
   Je me sens faible.
❏ My arms/legs are cramping.
   J'ai des crampes dans les bras/jambes.
❏ I have a headache.
   J'ai mal à la tête.
❏ My mouth is dry.
   J'ai la bouche sèche.
❏ I have fainted.
   Je me suis évanoui(e).
❏ My stomach is bloating.
   J'ai l'estomac ballonné.
❏ I feel lightheaded after standing up.
   J'ai la tête qui tourne lorsque je me relève.
❏ My heart races after a little bit of exertion.
   J'ai le cœur qui bat très vite au moindre effort.
❏ I've had these symptoms for____ hours/days.
   J'observe ces symptômes depuis ____heures/jours.

Fever

This section is designed to report information regarding fever. Fever is commonly associated with many illnesses. Use this section if you have fever, regardless of other associated medical problems such as cough, etc. The section also includes other complaints commonly associated with fever. It is in your best interest to review the following section and then complete any additional sections which may pertain to your medical problem. Refer to the Temperature Scale.

La fièvre

Cette section a été conçue pour fournir des renseignements concernant la fièvre. De nombreuses maladies sont souvent accompagnées de fièvre. Consultez cette section si vous avez de la fièvre, quels que soient les autres problèmes médicaux que vous puisssiez avoir, tel que la toux, etc. Cette section contient aussi d'autres symptômes communément associés à la fièvre. Il est dans votre intérêt de passer en revue la section suivante puis de compléter toute section supplémentaire pouvant concerner votre problème medical. Voir l'échelle de temperature.

Check only those questions to which you answer YES.
Cochez seulement les questions auxquelles vous répondez OUI.

Complaint
Symptômes
❑ I have a fever.
My fever began ＿＿ hours/days/weeks ago.
    J'ai de la fièvre.
        J'ai de la fièvre depuis ＿＿ heures/jours/semaines.

Associated symptoms and history:
Symptômes associés et informations complémentaires:
❑ I have chills
    J'ai des frissons.
❑ I have sweats.
    J'ai des suées.
❑ I have shaking chills that I cannot stop. These last about
    ＿＿＿minutes.

Quand je me mets à trembler, je ne peux pas m'arrêter.
❑ I have a headache.
    J'ai mal à la tête.
❑ I have chest pain. (Refer to Chest Pain Section)
    J'ai une douleur à la poitrine. (Voir section) douleur à la poitrine)
❑ I have a cough. (Refer to Cough Section)
    Je tousse. (Voir section toux)
❑ I have abdominal pain.(Refer to Abdominal Pain Section)
    J'ai une douleur abdominale. (Voir section douleur abdominale)
❑ I have pain when I urinate.(Refer to Urinary Tract Infection
    Section)
    Cela me fait mal quand j'urine. (Voir section infection des voies
        urinaire)
❑ I have diarrhea. (Refer to Diarrhea Section)
    J'ai la diarrhée. (Voir diarrhée)
❑ I have taken these medications.
      (Show medications)
    Voici les médicaments que j'ai pris.
      (Montrer ces médicaments)
❑ I have a rash.
    J'ai de l'urticaire.
❑ I have a stiff neck.
    J'ai une raideur dans la nuque.
❑ I have lost weight.
    J'ai perdu du poids.
❑ I have fatigue.
    Je me sens fatigué(e).
❑ I have malaise.
    J'ai des malaises.
❑ I am short of breath. (Refer to Pulmonary Section)
    Je suis essoufflé(e). (Voir la section pulmonaire)

Nausea

Nausea is an extremely common event, usually associated with vomiting. If you are vomiting please review and complete the vomiting
section as well.

This section, and others, will provide pertinent information to your physician regarding this problem.

La nausée

La nausée est un phénomène extrêment courant, généralement accompagné de vomissements. Si vous souffrez de vomissements, veuillez également consulter et compléter la section vomissements.

Cette section, ainsi que d'autres, fourniront des renseignements importants à votre médecin concernant votre problème.

Check only those questions to which you answer YES.
Cochez seulement les questions auxquelles vous répondez OUI.

Complaint
Symptômes
❏ I have nausea.
  J'ai la nausée.
❏ I have been nauseated for ____ minutes/hours/days.
  J'ai la nausée depuis ____ minutes/heures/jours.

Associated symptoms and history
Symptômes associés et informations complémentaires
❏ I have a cold.
  J'ai le rhume.
❏ I have been vomiting.
  J'ai des vomissements.
❏ I have a fever.
  J'ai de la fièvre.
❏ I have diarrhea.
  J'ai la diarrhée.
❏ I have been dizzy.
  J'ai des vertiges.
❏ The nausea is constant.
  J'ai la nausée en permanence.
❏ The nausea is intermittent.
  J'ai la nausée de façon intermittente.

❏ The nausea is associated with abdominal pain. (Refer to Abdominal Pain Section)

La nausée se combine à une douleur abdominale. (Voir section douleur abdominale)

❏ The nausea gets better when I vomit.

La nausée s'atténue lorsque je vomis.

❏ The nausea gets better when I move my bowels.

La nausée s'atténue lorsque je vais à la selle.

❏ I have been sweating profusely.

Je transpire abondamment.

Vomiting

Vomiting is not an uncommon problem. It is usually associated with another medical problem. Review your health status for the past several weeks. Inform your physician of any unusual problems. Review these questions carefully.

Les vomissements

Il n'est pas rare d'avoir des vomissements. Ceux-ci sont généralement liés à un autre problème médical. Faites le bilan de votre état de santé des dernières semaines. Si vous constatez un problème anormal, parlez-en à votre médecin. Considérez attentivement les questions suivantes.

Check only those questions to which you answer YES.
Cochez seulement les questions auxquelles vous répondez OUI.

Complaint
Symptômes
I have been vomiting.

J'ai des vomissements.

The problem started _____ minutes/hours/days ago.

Le problème a débuté il y a _____ minutes/hours/days ago.

Associated symptoms and history
Symptômes associés et informations complémentaires
The vomit has:

Quand je vomis, je vomis:

❏ red blood present. (Refer to Gastrointestinal Bleeding Section)

du sang rouge. (Voir la section du saignement gastrointestinal)

❏ black little flecks that look like coffee grounds.

des petites particules noires qui ressemblent à des grains de café.

❏ green material.

une substance verte.

❏ food I ate several hours ago.

ce que j'ai mangé plusieurs heures auparavant.

❏ food I ate at my last meal.

ce que j'ai mangé à mon dernier repas.

❏ I feel dehydrated.

Je me sens déshydraté(e).

❏ I get lightheaded when I stand up.

J'ai la tête qui tourne lorsque je me relève.

❏ I passed out.

Je me suis évanoui(e).

❏ My heart is pounding very hard.

J'ai le cœur qui bat très fort.

❏ My heart is racing.

J'ai le cœur qui bat à toute vitesse.

❏ I cannot keep anything down.

Je vomis tout ce que je mange.

❏ I have abdominal pain. (Refer to Abdominal Pain Section)

J'ai une douleur abdominale. (Voir section douleur abdominale)

❏ I have diarrhea. (Refer to Diarrhea Section)

J'ai la diarrhée. (Voir section diarrhée)

❏ I have had aches and pains in my muscles and joints.

J'ai des courbatures et des douleurs dans les muscles et les
articulations.

❏ I feel like I have a cold.

J'ai l'impression d'avoir le rhume.

❏ I have taken these medications. (Show medications)

J'ai pris ces médicaments. (Montrer ces médicaments)

❏ I have taken clear fluids.

Je n'ai consommé que des fluides clairs.

❏ I have been unable to keep anything down.

Je vomis tout ce que je mange.

Hives and Anaphylactic Shock

Hives are not an uncommon event. Hives present as raised areas which have a central area that appears normal. Usually, hives itch. The itching may be profound. The absence of itching is an important piece of information. If the hives are painful but not itchy, please be sure that the physician knows this piece of information. Anaphylactic shock is the development of an acute allergic reaction during which the airway may be obstructed and cardiovascular collapse (and death) may ensue. This section addresses both of these problems. If the patient is unable to answer these questions, please fill out as many of the questions as possible for him/her.

L'urticaire et les chocs anaphylactiques

L'urticaire n'est pas un phénomène rare. L'urticaire se présente sous la forme de boursouflures dont la partie centrale semble normale. Généralement, l'urticaire démange. La démangeaison peut être profonde. L'absence de démangeaison est une information importante. Veillez à le faire savoir à votre médecin. Un choc anaphylactique correspond au développement d'une réaction allergique aiguë durant laquelle les voies respiratoires peuvent être obstruées, résulatnt en un collapsus cardio-vasculaire entraînant la mort. Cette section traite de ces deux problèmes. Si le patient n'est pas en état de répondre à ces questions, veuillez compléter autant de questions que possible.

Check only those questions to which you answer YES.
Cochez seulement les questions auxquelles vous répondez OUI.

Complaint
Symptômes

❏ I have hives.

J'ai de l'urticaire.

❑ I have difficulty breathing.

   J'ai du mal à respirer.

❑ I cannot breath.

   Je n'arrive pas à respirer.

❑ I cannot swallow.

   Je n'arrive pas à avaler.

❑ I have passed out recently. It was _____ minutes/hours ago.

   Je me suis récemment évanoui(e). Il y a _____ minutes/heures.

❑ The problem began _____ hours/days ago.

   Ce problème a débuté il y a _____ heures/jours.

Associated symptoms and history

Symptômes associés et informations complémentaires

❑ The hives began very quickly.

   L'urticaire survient très vite.

❑ The hives come and go over several hours.

   L'urticaire apparaît et disparaît sur une période de plusieurs heures.

❑ The hives itch.

   L'urticaire me démange.

❑ The hives have been present for _____ days/weeks.

   J'ai de l'urticaire depuis _____ jours/semaines.

❑ The hives are painful but do not itch.

   L'urticaire me fait mal mais ne me démange pas.

   The area where I have had hives before has a residual dark color.
   (Show area of pigmentation)

   La zone où j'ai déjà eu de l'urticaire est restée sombre. (Montrer
   l'endroit de la pigmentation)

❑ I have been taking a new medication. (Include both prescription
   and non-prescription medications and any recreational drugs)

   Je prends un nouveau medicament. (Cela vaut à la fois pour les
   médicaments prescrits par ordonance et pour ceux en vente libre.
   Faire figurer aussi les drogues douces)

❑ I am taking the following medications. (Refer to Medication
   Section)

   Je prends les médicaments suivants. (Voir la section médicaments)

❏ I have recently started on an antibiotic. (Show the antibiotic)
J'ai commencé récemment à prendre un antibiotique. (Montrer cet antibiotique)

❏ I have been exposed to animal saliva.
J'ai été en contact avec de la salive animale.

❏ I have been exposed to plants.
J'ai été en contact avec des plantes.

❏ I have been exposed to raw fish.
J'ai été en contact avec du poisson cru.

❏ I have been exposed to vegetables.
J'ai été en contact avec des légumes.

❏ I have been exposed to latex.
J'ai été en contact avec du latex.

❏ I have been exposed to new metals.
J'ai été en contact avec des métaux.

❏ I have been stung by a bee/wasp/hornet.
Je me suis fait piquer par une abeille/une guêpe/un frelon.

❏ I have environmental allergies.
Je souffre d'allergies liées à l'environnement.

❏ The hives usually occur within 30 minutes of eating. (Review your dietary history looking for fish, shellfish, nuts, peanuts, soy, wheat, milk, and eggs.)
L'urticaire survient généralement dans les 30 minutes qui suivent un repas. (Passez en revue ce que vous avez mangé récemment en recherchant particulièrement les poissons, les crustacés, les noix, les cacahuètes, le soja, le blé, les œufs et le lait.)

❏ I have a fever.
J'ai de la fièvre.

❏ I have a viral syndrome.
J'ai un syndrome viral.

❏ I have been exposed to cold temperatures.
J'ai été exposé(e) à des températures très froides.

❏ I have had a weight loss. I have lost _____ lb/kg.
(2.2 pounds = 1 kilogram)
J'ai perdu du poids. J'ai perdu _____ lb/kg.

❏ I have joint pain.

    J'ai des douleurs articulaires.

❏ I have muscle pains.

    J'ai des douleurs musculaires.

❏ I have heat intolerance.

    Je ne supporte pas la chaleur.

❏ I have cold intolerance.

    Je ne supporte pas le froid.

❏ I have abdominal pain. (Refer to Abdominal Pain Section)

    J'ai des douleurs abdominales. (Voir la section concernant les douleurs abdominales)

❏ I have an allergy to aspirin.

    Je suis allergique à l'aspirine.

❏ I have an allergy to radiographic contrast.

    Je suis allergique aux produits de contraste radiographique.

❏ I have an allergy to iodine.

    Je suis allergique à l'iode.

❏ I have had a recent injection. The injection was on _____ day/month/year. (Show what was injected and explain why.)

    J'ai eu une piqûre récemment. La piqûre a eu lieu _____ jour/mois/année. (Indiquer la nature de la piqûre et sa raison d'être.)

❏ I have had anaphylactic shock in the past. This occurred on _____. (date)

    J'ai déjà eu un choc anaphylactique. Cela s'est produit _____. (date)

❏ I am allergic to bees.

    Je suis allergique aux abeilles.

❏ I have been eating Chinese food recently.

    J'ai magé de la nourriture chinoise récemment.

❏ I have been eating fish recently.

    J'ai mangé du poisson récemment.

❏ I am taking isoniazide.

    Je prends de l'isoniazide.

Headache

Headaches are quite common. Many times the headache has been evaluated prior to leaving the United States for a trip abroad. The information and studies which have been performed are very useful for a new physician during an assessment. Please think through the studies which have been performed in the past and record them in the front of the book. Please review the Table of Contents and fill out any associated sections. The Visual Field Diagram may be useful.

Les maux de tête

Les maux de tête sont très courants. Très souvent, ces maux de tête ont déjà été diagnostiqués par un médecin aux Etats-Unis avant le départ pour un voyage à l'étranger. Veuillez vous remémorer les examens qui ont été faits par le passé et les noter en début de livre.

Check only those questions to which you answer YES.
Cochez seulement les questions auxquelles vous répondez OUI.

Complaint
Symptômes
❑ I have a headache.
 J'ai mal à la tête.
❑ The pain is here. (Demonstrate)
 J'ai mal là. (Démontrer)
❑ The headache began about ____ minutes/hours/days/weeks ago.
 Mon mal de tête a débuté il y a ____ minutes/heures/jours/
 semaines.
❑ The headache started suddenly/slowly.
 Mon mal de tête a débuté soudainement/lentement.
❑ The pain is severe. (Refer to Visual Pain Scale)
 La douleur est intense. (Voir echelle de douleur)

Associated symptoms and history
Symptômes associés et informations complémentaires
❑ This the first time I have had a headache this severe.
 C'est la première fois que j'ai un mal de tête aussi violent.

❏ This is the worst headache of my life.
Je n'ai jamais eu un mal de tête pareil.
❏ The pain: (check all that apply)
La douleur: (cochez ce qui convient)
  ❏ is on one side of my head.
  se situe sur un côté de la tête.
  ❏ is on both sides of my head.
  se situe des deux côtés de la tête.
  ❏ is pulsating or throbbing.
  élance.
  ❏ is a pressure or tight sensation.
  me comprime la tête.
❏ began suddenly and increased in severity quite quickly.
a débuté soudainement et s'est accrue très vite.
❏ is deep inside my head.
est logée en profondeur.
❏ is continuous.
est continue.
❏ aggravated by routine physical activity.
s'accentue lorsque j'ai une activité physique normale.
❏ The pain radiates into my neck. (Demonstrate)
La douleur s'étend à la nuque. (Démontrer)
❏ I prefer to rest in a quiet room.
Je préfère me reposer dans une chambre calme.
❏ I have had trauma to my head. The problem started _____
minutes/hours/days ago.
J'ai eu un traumatisme crânien. Le problème a débuté il y a _____
minutes/heures/jours.
❏ I can remain active and do not need to rest because of the headache.
Je peux continuer mes activités et n'ai pas besoin de me reposer
à cause de mon mal de tête.
❏ I have nausea.
J'ai la nausée.
❏ I have vomiting.
J'ai des vomissements.

❏ I do not like bright lights.
Je ne supporte pas les fortes lumières.
❏ I do not like loud sounds.
Je ne supporte les bruits forts.
❏ I have seen flashing lights.
Je vois des éclairs lumineux.
❏ I have had tearing from the eye on the same side as my headache.
J'ai une sensation de déchirure qui part de l'œil situé du même
   côté que mon mal de tête.
❏ I have had red eyes.
J'ai les yeux rouges.
❏ I have a stuffy nose.
J'ai le nez pris.
❏ I have had sweating.
J'ai des suées.
❏ I have had a fever. (Refer to Temperature Scale)
J'ai de la fièvre. (Voir l'échelle de température)
❏ I have had a cough.
Je tousse.
❏ I am having my normal menstrual period.
J'ai mes règles normalement.
❏ I am taking hormone replacement therapy.
Je prends des hormones de substitution.
I started having the headache just after:
Mon mal de tête a débuté juste après:
   ❏ seeing flickering lights.
     que j'ai vu des lumières vacillantes.
   ❏ seeing a strong, bright light.
     que j'ai vu une lumière forte et vive.
   ❏ experiencing a foul smell.
     que j'ai senti une mauvaise odeur.
   ❏ hearing very loud noises.
     que j'ai entendu des bruits très violents.
❏ I have been under a great deal of stress.
Je suis très stressé(e).

❏ I have been traveling through different time zones.
J'ai plusieurs fuseaux horaire de décalage.
❏ I have been experiencing altitude changes.
J'ai changé d'altitude.
❏ I have been dieting.
Je suis au régime.
❏ I have been having irregular sleeping patterns.
Mon sommeil n'est pas régulier.

Previous treatments
Traitements antérieurs
❏ I I have taken these medications. (Show medications)
J'ai pris ces médicaments-ci. (Montrer ces médicaments)
❏ I I have taken my usual medication for this problem. (Refer to
Medication Section)
J'ai pris mes médicaments habituels pour ce problème. (Voir
section médicaments)

Previous history of headaches
Antécédents concernant vos maux de tête
❏ I have had migraine headaches in the past.
J'ai déjà eu des migraines.
❏ I have had tension headaches in the past.
J'ai déjà eu des maux de tête dûs à la tension nerveuse.
❏ I have had cluster headaches in the past.
J'ai déjà eu des maux de tête en série.
❏ I have had a complete neurological evaluation in the past for these
headaches.
J'ai déjà eu un bilan neurologique complet pour ces maux de tête.
❏ The symptoms I have now are the same as before. They have not
changed.
Les symptômes de cette fois-ci sont les mêmes que ceux des fois
antérieures. Les symptômes n'ont pas changé.

Seizures

Travelers with a history of seizures should inform their companion of the diagnosis. The front section of this book should be filled out completely and any further pertinent information from their personal physician located in a readily accessible and well known place during their travels. Please review the Table of Contents and fill out any associated sections. The Visual Field Diagram may be useful.

A note to companions: The occurrence of seizures is usually associated with loss of consciousness and development of a state of confusion after resolution of the seizure. This post seizure state of confusion is called the post-ictal state. The individual who has the seizure is unable to provide accurate information to his/her companions. In this event, the pertinent medical history is obtained from the companions or observers of the seizure event. A description of the seizure is important since it relates features that will assist a foreign healthcare provider with important information regarding the event, its cause, and the treatment. An accurate description of the event is essential to providing the patient optimal care.

The information below is designed to provide the OBSERVER of the seizure with information that will be useful to a foreign health care provider. The patient should inform the health care provider of any additional information after the post-ictal state has resolved.

If the patient is able to provide further information, this section should be reviewed with the patient and the observer together. The more information you provide, the better the decision. If you feel it might benefit your health, answer more than one section.

Les attaques cérébrales

Un voyageur ayant déjà fait une ou plusieurs attaque(s) cérébrale(s) doit absolument en informer son compagnon/sa compagne de voyage, compléter soigneusement la section de garde de ce livre, et garder tout autre renseignement important fourni par son médecin personnel dans un endroit connu de tous et facile d'accès pendant toute la durée du voyage.

Notice à l'usage des compagnons de voyage: Lorsque survient une attaque, celle-ci s'accompagne généralement d'une perte de conscience ainsi que d'un état confus après la fin de l'attaque. Cet état confus s'appelle état post-ictal. L'individu qui fait une attaque n'est pas en mesure de fournir à ses compagnons des renseignments précis. Dans ce cas, ce sont ses compagnons de voyage ou les personnes qui ont assisté à l'attaque qui peuvent expliquer précisément ce qui s'est passé. Il est important de décrire l'attaque car cette description met en évidence des caractéristiques qui fourniront au praticien étranger des renseignements très utiles sur l'attaque, sa cause et son traitement. Une description précise de l'événement est essentielle pour garantir un traitement optimal.

Les informations ci-dessous concernent LA PERSONNE QUI A ASSISTE à l'attaque. Cette section a été conçue pour fournir à la personne ayant assisté à l'attaque des informations qui seront utiles au pratitien étranger. Le patient devra fournir au praticien tout information supplémentaire une fois que le stade post-ictal sera terminé.

Si le patient est en mesure de fournir des renseignements supplémentaires, il devra, avec l'aide de la personne ayant assisté à l'attaque, passer cette section en revue. Plus les renseignements fournis seront nombreux, meilleure sera la décision prise par le praticien. Si vous pensez que cela peut être dans l'intérêt de votre santé, ne vous limitez pas à une section, complétez-en plusieurs.

Check only those questions to which you answer YES.
Cochez seulement les questions auxquelles vous répondez OUI.

Complaint
Symptômes
❏ I/my companion has had a seizure.
    J'ai eu/mon compagnon (ma compagne) a fait une attaque.
❏ The seizure occurred approximately _____ minutes/hours ago.
    L'attaque s'est produite il y a environ _____ minutes/heures.

Associated symptoms and history:
Symptômes associés et informations complémentaires:
❏ The seizure lasted _____ minutes.
    L'attaque a duré _____ minutes.

❏ I observed that the patient: (choose all that apply)
J'ai constaté que le patient: (choisissez ce qui convient)
❏ was staring into space.
   fixait le vide.
❏ was smacking his/her lips.
   claquait des lèvres.
❏ was blinking his/her eyes repeatedly.
   clignait des yeux de façon répétée.
❏ complained that an "aura" was present just before the event
     occurred.
   s'est plaint de la présence d'une "aura" juste avant l'événement.
❏ was breathing heavily.
   respirait fort.
❏ was confused.
   avait l'esprit troublé
❏ was drooling.
   bavait.
❏ was dizzy.
   avait des vertiges.
❏ had his/her eyes roll up into the back of his/her head.
   avait les yeux révulsés.
❏ fell down.
   était tombé par terre.
❏ was unable to move.
   ne pouvait plus bouger.
❏ was talking with difficulty.
   parlait avec difficulté.
❏ was biting his/her tongue.
   se mordait la langue.
❏ was complaining of a tingling sensation.
     (Observer should describe where.)
   se plaignait de picotements.
     (L'observateur doit décrire à quel endroit.)
❏ was stomping his/her foot.
   marchait lourdement.
❏ was waving his/her hands.

agitait les mains.

❏ had an abrupt loss of consciousness.

avait soudain perdu connaissance.

❏ had stiffening of the muscles.

avait les muscles qui se raidissaient.

❏ had muscle jerking.

avait les muscles qui se contractaient.

❏ struck his/her head.

s'était cogné la tête.

❏ appeared to be awake but was not in contact with the rest of the world.

semblait éveillé mais n'était pas en contact avec le reste du monde.

❏ I observed that the patient had repeated: (choose all that apply)

J'ai constaté que le patient ne cessait de: (choisissez ce qui convient)

❏ facial grimaces.

aire des grimaces.

❏ chewing.

mâcher.

❏ lip smacking.

claquer des lèvres.

❏ snapping fingers.

claquer des doigts.

❏ words or phrases.

répéter les mêmes mots ou la même phrase.

❏ The patient was hostile when I tried to restrain him/her.

Le patient était agressif quand j'essayais de l'empêcher de le faire.

❏ After the seizure, the patient was confused and acted like she/he did not know where he/she was.

Après son attaque, le patient avait l'esprit troublé. On aurait dit qu'il/elle ne savait pas où il/elle était.

❏ The patient defecated (had an involuntary bowel movement) during or after the seizure.

Le patient a déféqué (est allé à la selle involontairement) pendant ou après son attaque.
❑ The patient urinated during or after the seizure.
Le patient a uriné pendant ou après son attaque.
❑ The patient dropped to the ground. It was like he/she lost all muscle control. I saw no jerking of the limbs.
Le patient est tombé à terre. On aurait dit qu'il/elle avait perdu tout contrôle de ses muscles. Je n'ai pas constaté que les membres se contractaient.
❑ The patient had an abrupt loss of consciousness. Just before this happened he/she screamed for no reason at all. The legs, back, and arms then became stiff. Next, the patient began to turn blue. Shortly after this, his/her legs, arms, and body began to jerk uncontrollably.
On voyait une bave mousseuse dans sa bouche. Cette mousse ne contenait pas de sang. Lorsque les contractions des membres ont cessé, le patient a commencé à respirer profondément et a semblé se détendre. Quand il a repris connaissance, le patient s'est plaint d'un mal de tête.
❑ A frothy sputum was seen in his/her mouth. This sputum did/did not (circle one) have blood. After the jerking stopped, the patient began to breathe deeply and appeared to relax. When he/she woke up the patient complained of a headache.
Le patient a soudain perdu connaissance. Juste avant que cela ne se produise, il/elle s'est mis à crier sans raison. Ses jambes, son dos et ses bras se sont alors raidis. Puis la patient est devenu bleu. Peu de temps après, ses jambes, ses bras et son corps se sont mis à se contracter de façon incontrôlée.
❑ The patient has had seizures in the past.
Le patient a déjà eu des attaques cérébrales.
❑ I have a diagnosis:
J'ai un diagnostic pour ces attaques:
  ❑ partial seizures.
  attaques partielles.
  ❑ simple partial seizures (aura).

attaques partielles simples (aura).
- ❏ complex partial seizures.
  attaques partielles complexes.
- ❏ atonic seizures.
  attaques atoniques.
- ❏ generalized seizures.
  attaques généralisées.
- ❏ convulsive type.
  de type convulsif.
- ❏ non-convulsive type.
  de type non-convulsif.
- ❏ I have epilepsy.
  Je fais des crises d'épilepsie.
- ❏ I have seizures but do not know what type of seizure disorder.
  Je fais des attaques mais je ne sais pas de quel type d'attaque je souffre.
- ❏ I have diabetes.
  J'ai du diabète.
- ❏ I take pills to control my diabetes. (Refer to Medication Section)
  Je prends des comprimés pour mon diabète. (Voir section médicaments)
- ❏ I take insulin for my diabetes.
  Je prends de l'insuline pour mon diabète.
- ❏ The patient has had recent head trauma.
  Le patient a récemment eu un traumatisme crânien.
- ❏ The patient has had a stroke recently.
  Le patient a récemment fait une crise cardiaque.
- ❏ The patient has a history of alcohol abuse.
  Le patient a un passé de dépendance à l'alcool.
- ❏ The patient has a history of drug abuse.
  Le patient a un passé de dépendance à la drogue.
- ❏ The patient has been using drugs recently.
  Le patient a récemment consommé de la drogue.
- ❏ The patient has a history of infection in the brain.
  Il y a eu beaucoup d'infections du cerveau dans la famille du patient.

❏ The patient has a family history of seizures.
Il y a eu beaucoup d'attaques dans la famille du patient.
❏ The patient has a history of:
Le patient a déjà eu à plusieurs reprises:
  ❏ low thyroid (hypothyroidism).
    un taux de sécrétions thyroïdiennes bas (hypothyroïdie).
  ❏ elevated thyroid (hyperthyroidism).
    un taux de sécrétions thyroïdiennes élévé (hyperthyroïdie).
  ❏ low blood sugars (hypoglycemia).
    un taux peu élevé de sucres dans le sang (hypoglycémie).
  ❏ kidney disease.
    une maladie des reins.
  ❏ recent surgery.
    une opération récente.
  ❏ porphyria.
    une porphyrie.
  ❏ cardiac arrest.
    un arrêt cardiaque.
  ❏ problems with the valves of the heart.
    des problèmes de valves cardiaques.
  ❏ HIV infection.
    une infection par le virus HIV.
  ❏ a tumor.
    une tumeur.
  ❏ blood clots.
    des caillots sanguins.
  ❏ psychiatric disorders.
    des troubles psychiatriques.

Dizziness

This section is designed to report information regarding dizziness. Dizziness refers to balance problems. The causes of dizziness are many and may be complicated or simple. The term vertigo is used in medical parlance for dizziness. The term dizziness means many things to many people. Often it may be a very vague and poorly defined complaint. Sometimes patients choose the term dizzy because their complaints are unusual and this is the closest term to that which they feel is applicable. Please characterize the problem as accurately as possible. The following section is designed to assist you with informing a physician of the complaint of the current problem. Review the questions before responding. Consider the events which you have experienced carefully.

Les vertiges

Cette section a été conçue pour fournir des renseignements sur les vertiges. Les vertiges sont liés à des problèmes d'équilibre. Il y a de nombreuses causes de vertige, et ces causes peuvent être compliquées ou simples. Dans le vocabulaire médical anglais, on utilise le terme vertigo pour faire référence aux vertiges. En fonction des personnes, le terme vertige recouvre des notions différentes. Souvent, les patients restent vagues et ont du mal à définir ce dont ils souffrent. Il arrive que les patients choisissent le terme vertige parce qu'ils n'ont pas l'habitude de ces symptômes et que le terme vertige leur semble être ce qui correspond le plus à leur problème. Veuillez essayer de décrire le problème de façon aussi précise que possible. La section suivante a été conçue pour vous aider à donner des renseignements au médecin sur le problème dont vous souffrez. Passez en revue les questions avant d'y répondre. Réfléchissez bien à ce que vous avez ressenti.

Check only those questions to which you answer YES.
Cochez seulement les questions auxquelles vous répondez OUI.

Complaint
Symptômes
❏ I feel dizzy.
    J'ai des vertiges.
❏ I have been dizzy for _____ minutes/hours/days.
    J'ai des vertiges depuis _____ minutes/heures/jours.
❏ I have a fever. (Refer to Temperature Scale)
    J'ai de la fièvre. (Voir l'échelle de température)

Associated symptoms and history
Symptômes associés et informations complémentaires

❏ The problems last for _____ minutes/hours.
   Ces problèmes durent pendant _____ minutes/heures.
❏ Dizziness comes and goes.
   Ces vertiges vont et viennent.
❏ I feel like I am spinning around in a room.
   J'ai l'impression de tourner come une toupie dans une pièce.
❏ I feel like the room is spinning around me.
   J'ai l'impression que la pièce tourne comme une toupie autour
   de moi.
❏ I am dizzy when I sit still.
   J'ai des vertiges même quand je suis assis(e) sans bouger.
❏ I feel lightheaded.
   J'ai la tête qui tourne.
❏ I feel faint.
   J'ai l'impression que je vais m'évanouir.
❏ I feel like I am floating.
   J'ai l'impression de flotter.
❏ I feel like I am not balanced.
   J'ai l'impression de ne pas avoir d'équilibre.
❏ I have passed out.
   Je me suis évanoui(e).
❏ I have a headache.
   J'ai mal à la tête.
❏ I have had seizures. (Refer to Seizure Section)
   J'ai déjà fait des attaques. (Voir section attaques cérébrales)
❏ The episodes are severe.
   Les crises sont violentes.
❏ The episodes are getting worse.
   Les crises sont de plus en plus violentes.
❏ The episodes are worse when I move.
   Les crises sont plus violentes lorsque je bouge.
❏ The surroundings tend to bob up and down when I move my head.
   Tout oscille autour de moi quand je bouge la tête.
❏ I recently had head trauma. (Refer to Head Diagrams)
   J'ai récemment eu un traumatisme crânien. (Voir les diagrammes
   de la tête)

❏ I have had a cold recently.
   J'ai eu un rhume récemment.
❏ I have had pain in the right/left/both ears.
   J'ai eu mal à l'oreille droite/gauche/aux deux oreilles.
❏ I have ringing in my ears.
   J'ai une sonnerie dans les oreilles.
❏ I have hearing loss on the right/left/both side(s).
   J'entends moins bien à droite/à gauche/des deux côtés.
❏ I have increased hearing loss when I turn my head like this.
   (Perform the motion)
   J'entends de moins en moins bien quand je tourne la tête comme
   cela. (Faire le mouvement)
❏ I have double vision.
   Je vois double.
❏ I have difficulty speaking.
   J'ai du mal à parler.
❏ I am anxious.
   Je suis angoissé(e)
❏ I have nausea.
   J'ai la nausée.
❏ I have been vomiting.
   J'ai des vomissements.
❏ I have difficulty walking.
   J'ai du mal à marcher.
❏ I am having chest pain. (Refer to Cardiac Section)
   J'ai une douleur dans la poitrine. (Voir section cardiologie)
❏ I have had this problem before. (Refer to Medical History Section)
   J'ai déjà eu ce problème. (Voir antécedents médicaux)
❏ I am having palpitations. (Refer to Cardiac Section)
   J'ai des palpitations. (Voir section cardiologie)

Stroke

Stroke (cerebrovascular accident) is an acute neurologic insult that
may be related to either insufficient blood flow or blood clots to a
specific section of the brain. The following questions will assist in
providing pertinent information to your physician regarding this

problem. The questions below may need to be answered by a friend or companion. Please be as objective regarding the events as possible. Answer all of the questions, if possible. Circle any appropriate answers within the sentences themselves. Please review the Table of Contents and fill out any associated sections. The Visual Field Diagram may be useful.

Les attaquaes d'apoplexie

L'attaque d'apoplexie (accident cérébro-vasculaire) est un problème neurologique grave qui peut être lié soit à une circulation sanguine insuffisante, soit à des caillots de sang dans une section spécifique du cerveau. Les questions suivantes aideront à fournir des renseignements importants à votre médecin concernant ce problème.

Il se peut qu'un(e) ami(e) ou un(e) compagnon/compagne ait à répondre aux questions ci-dessous. Veuillez relater les événements de façon aussi objective que possible. Répondez aux questions dans la mesure du possible. A l'intérieur des phrases proposées, entourez toute réponse qui vous paraît pertinente.

Check only those questions to which you answer YES.
Cochez seulement les questions auxquelles vous répondez OUI.

Complaint
Symptômes
❑ I/my partner may have had a stroke.
   J'ai fait/Mon partenaire a fait une attaque d'apoplexie.
❑ This problem occurred _____ minutes/hours ago.
   Ce problème s'est produit il y a _____ minutes/heures.

Associated symptoms and history
Symptômes associés et informations complémentaires
❑ My face is weak/numb on the right/left side.
   Le côté droit/gauche de mon visage est mou/paralysé.
❑ My right/left arm is weak/numb.
   Mon bras droit/gauche est mou/n'a plus de sensations.
❑ My right/left leg is weak/numb.
   Ma jambe droite/gauche est molle/n'a plus de sensations.
❑ I am having difficulty speaking.

J'ai du mal à parler.

❑ I am having difficulty swallowing.

J'ai du mal à avaler.

❑ I cough when I try to swallow liquids.

Je tousse quand j'essaie d'avaler des liquides.

❑ I have trouble understanding written/spoken/both words.

J'ai du mal à comprendre les mots que je lis/que j'entends/les deux.

❑ I have been having trouble walking since this problem began.

J'ai du mal à marcher depuis que ce problème a commencé.

❑ I have a headache. (Complete the Headache Section)

J'ai mal à la tête. (Compléter la section maux de tête)

❑ I cannot stand up. I keep losing my balance.

Je ne peux pas me tenir debout. Je perds l'équilibre.

❑ I have had a stroke in the past. This occurred on
_____ (date).

J'ai déjà fait une attaque d'apoplexie. Cela s'est produit il y a
_____ (date).

❑ I have been on medications for this problem.
(Refer to Medication Section)

Je prends des médicaments pour ce problème.
(Voir section médicaments)

❑ I have a history of seizures.

J'ai déjà fait plusieurs attaques.

❑ I have hypertension.

Je fais de l'hypertension.

❑ I have diabetes.

J'ai du diabète.

❑ I have problems with the valves of my heart.

J'ai un problème de valve cardiaque.

❑ I have vascular disease.

J'ai une maladie vasculaire.

❑ I have multiple sclerosis.

J'ai la sclérose en plaques.

❑ I have been using blood thinners.

Je prends des anticoagulants.

Dental Pain

Toothaches or injury can be common during travel. Injury is usually quite obvious. Tooth pain can be caused by a dental infection. It also may be due to a sinus problem and not a tooth problem. Atmospheric pressure can cause pain as with flying, hiking in the mountains, or underwater diving. A gum infection may need to be drained or may need antibiotics.

Le mal de dents

Avoir mal aux dents ou se faire mal aux dents arrive fréquememnt en voyage. Il est facile de savoir comment on s'est fait mal aux dents. Le mal de dents, en revanche, peut être causé par une infection dentaire. Il peut aussi être dû à un problème de sinus, et non à un problème de dents. La pression atmosphérique lorsque l'on est en avion, que l'on fait du vélo en montagne ou de la plongée sous-marine peut aussi causer des douleurs dentaires. Une infection des gencives peut nécessiter un drainage ou des antibiotiques.

Check only those questions to which you answer YES.
Cochez seulement les questions auxquelles vous répondez OUI.

Complaint
Symptômes

❏ I have a problem with my tooth/teeth.
  J'ai un problème à une dent/aux dents.
❏ I have a fever. (Refer to Temperature Scale)
  J'ai de la fièvre. (Voir l'échelle de temperature)
❏ I have a broken tooth.
  J'ai une dent cassée.
❏ I have no injury.
  Je n'ai pas de blessure.
❏ I have an injury. (Demonstrate)
  J'ai une blessure. (Démontrer)
❏ I have an infection in my lip.
  J'ai une infection à la lèvre.
❏ I have an infection in my gums.
  J'ai une infection à la gencive.

❏ I have bleeding coming from my gums.
  Je saigne des gencives.
❏ This started _____ minutes/hours/days ago.
  Cela a débuté il y a _____ minutes/heures/jours.

Associated symptoms and history
Symptômes associés et informations complémentaires
❏ I have pain. (Refer to Pain Scale)
  J'ai mal. (Voir echelle de douleur)
❏ The pain is:
  La douleur est:
  ❏ throbbing.
    lancinante.
  ❏ dull.
    sourde.
  ❏ sharp.
    aiguë.
  ❏ intermittent.
    intermittente.
  ❏ constant.
    constante.
❏ I have a cold.
  J'ai le rhume.
❏ I have a current sinus problem.
  J'ai un problème aux sinus en ce moment.
❏ I am nauseated.
  J'ai la nausée.
❏ I have a fever. (Refer to Fever Section)
  J'ai de la fièvre. (Voir section fièvre)
❏ I have a headache. (Refer to Headache Section)
  J'ai mal à la tête. (Voir section mal à la tête)
❏ I have been underwater diving (scuba or snorkeling).
  J'ai fait de la plongée sous-marine (plongée bouteille ou masque
  et tuba).
❏ I have been traveling on airplanes.
  J'ai voyagé par avion.

❑ I have been in the mountains.

Je suis allé(e) en montagne.

❑ I have taken medications. (Show medications)

J'ai pris ces médicaments-ci. (Montrer les médicaments)

❑ This has never happened before.

Cela ne m'est jamais arrivé.

❑ This has happened before, _____ days/months/years ago.

Cela m'est déjà arrive, il y a _____ jours/mois/ans.

Ear Problems or Hearing Loss

Ear pain is usually due to an infection or trauma. Infections can be due to a bacteria (treated with antibiotics) or a virus (which resolves by itself and is treated with medications to improve the symptoms). The infection is usually behind the ear drum. An infection can be in the ear canal and is often caused by swimming (swimmer's ear). Pressure on the ear from flying, underwater diving, or travel to the mountains can cause pressure trauma to the ear. The ear can even rupture. Something in the ear can cause pain.

Hearing loss is usually due to infection or trauma. Wax that blocks the ear can cause hearing loss. Ringing, buzzing, popping, or clicking can be caused by infection or trauma but may be due to a nerve problem.

Les problèmes d'oreille ou les pertes d'audition

Les douleurs à l'oreille sont généralement dues à une infection ou à un traumatisme. Les infections peuvent être dues à une bactérie (on les traite alors avec des antibiotiques) ou à un virus (qui se résoud de lui-même et qu'on traite avec des médicaments pour soulager les symptômes). L'infection se situe généralement derrière le tympan de l'oreille. Une infection peut se loger dans le canal auditif et est souvent causée par la natation (l'oreille du nageur). La pression qui s'exerce sur l'oreille quand on est en avion, qu'on fait de la plongée sous-marine et qu'on voyage en montagne peut causer un traumatisme à l'oreille. Le tympan de l'oreille peut même éclater. Quelque chose à l'intérieur de l'oreille peut aussi causer une douleur.

Une perte d'audition est généralement due à une infection ou à un traumatisme. Elle peut aussi être causée par de la cire qui bouche l'oreille. Les bruits de sonnerie, les vrombissements, les bruits de détonation ou les claquements peuvent être causés par une infection ou un traumatisme mais peuvent être aussi dûs à un problème de nerfs.

Check only those questions to which you answer YES.
Cochez seulement les questions auxquelles vous répondez OUI.

Complaint
Symptômes

❏ I have a problem with my ear. (right/left/both)
  J'ai un problème à l'oreille. (droite/gauche/aux deux oreilles)
❏ I have pain in my ear. (right/left/both)
  J'ai mal à l'oreille. (droite/gauche/aux deux oreilles)
❏ I have no injury.
  Je n'ai pas de blessure.
❏ I have an injury. (Demonstrate)
  J'ai une blessure. (Démontrer)
❏ I have a new hearing problem. (left/right/both)
  Je n'entends pas bien de l'oreille droite/gauche/des deux oreilles, et c'est nouveau.
❏ I cannot hear at all.
  Je n'entends rien du tout.
❏ My hearing has decreased.
  J'entends moins bien qu'avant.
❏ I hear ringing.
  J'ai une sonnerie dans l'oreille.
❏ I hear buzzing.
  J'ai une vibration dans l'oreille.
❏ I hear popping or clicking.
  J'entends des claquements et des bruits de détonation.
❏ I have something in my ear.
  J'ai quelque chose dans l'oreille.
❏ This started _____ minutes/hours/days ago.
  Cela a débuté il y a _____ minutes/heures/jours.

Associated symptoms and history
Symptômes associés et informations complémentaires

❏ I have pain. (Refer to Visual Pain Scale and Head Diagram)
J'ai mal. (Voir echelle de douleur et le diagramme de la tête)

❏ The pain is:
La douleur est:

  ❏ throbbing.
    lancinante.

  ❏ dull.
    sourde.

  ❏ sharp.
    aiguë.

  ❏ intermittent.
    intermittente.

  ❏ constant.
    constante.

❏ I have a cold.
J'ai le rhume.

❏ I have a current sinus problem.
J'ai un problème aux sinus en ce moment.

❏ I am nauseated. (Refer to Nausea Section)
J'ai la nausée. (Voir section nausée)

❏ I have a fever. (Refer to Fever Section)
J'ai de la fièvre. (Voir section fièvre)

❏ I have a headache. (Refer to Headache Section)
J'ai mal à la tête. (Voir section mal à la tête)

❏ I have a toothache.
J'ai mal aux dents.

❏ I have decreased hearing in my affected ear.
J'entends moins bien de l'oreille affectée.

❏ I have drainage coming from my ear. The drainage is:
J'ai l'oreille qui coule. La substance est:

  ❏ clear.
    clair.

  ❏ green.
    verte.

❏ yellowish.
  jaunâtre.
❏ bloody.
  contient du sang.
❏ I have been exposed to very loud noises.
  J'ai été en contact avec des bruits très forts.
❏ I have been swimming.
  Je me suis baigné(e).
❏ I have been underwater diving (scuba or snorkeling).
  J'ai fait de la plongée sous-marine (plongée bouteille ou masque
  et tuba).
❏ I have been traveling on airplanes.
  J'ai voyagé par avion.
❏ I have been in the mountains.
  Je suis allé(e) en montagne.
❏ Please look at my medical history.
  Veuillez consulter mes antécédents médicaux.
❏ I have used ear drops.
  J'ai pris des gouttes pour les oreilles.
❏ I have taken medications.
  J'ai pris des médicaments.
❏ This has never happened before.
  Cela ne m'est jamais arrive.
❏ This has happened before, _____ days/years ago.
  Cela m'est déjà arrivé il y a _____ jours/ans.
❏ I have no prior ear problems.
  Je n'ai jamais eu de problème à l'oreille.
❏ I wear hearing aids.
  Je porte un appareil auditif.
❏ I use medications for my ears. (Show medications)
  Je prends des médicaments pour les oreilles. (Montrer les
  medicaments)

Eye Problem or Visual loss—No Trauma

The development of ocular problems can be associated with trauma
or there can be non-traumatic causes. In some cases, both may be

present, such as an individual with previous eye disease who has been involved in a motor vehicle accident.

A review of both the trauma section for eye injury and this section may be best for individuals who are unsure of their problems. Please review the Table of Contents and fill out any associated sections. The Visual Field Diagram may be useful.

Les problèmes à l'œil ou les pertes de vision —sans traumatisme
Le développement de troubles oculaires peut être lié à des causes traumatiques ou non traumatiques. Dans certains cas, les deux peuvent co-exister, comme dans le cas d'un individu ayant déjà une maladie de l'œil et étant victime d'un accident de la circulation.

Il serait bon que les personnes n'étant pas sûres de ce dont elles souffrent consultent à la fois la section sur les traumatismes et cette section-ci.

Check only those questions to which you answer YES.
Cochez seulement les questions auxquelles vous répondez OUI.

Complaint
Symptômes
❑ I have a problem with my eye. (right/left/both)
    J'ai un problème à l'œil. (droit/gauche/aux deux)
❑ I have a problem with my eyelid. (right/left/both)
    J'ai un problème à la paupière. (droite/gauche/aux deux)
❑ I have problem with my vision. (right/left/both)
    J'ai un problème de vue. (à l'œil droit/gauche/aux deux yeux)
❑ I cannot see at all.
    Je ne vois rien du tout.
❑ Part of my vision is gone. (left/right) (top/bottom)
    J'ai perdu une partie de ma vision. (à gauche/à droite)
      (en haut/en bas)
❑ My vision is blurred.
    Je vois flou.
❑ I see stars or flashes.
    Je vois des étoiles ou des éclairs.
❑ This happened _____ minutes/hours/days ago.
    Cela s'est passé il y a _____ minutes/heures/jours.

Associated symptoms and history

Symptômes associés et informations complémentaires

❑ My eye is red.

　J'ai l'œil rouge.

❑ I have drainage from the eye. It is:

　J'ai l'œil qui coule. Cette substance est:

　　❑ clear.

　　clair.

　　❑ yellow.

　　jaune.

❑ My eyelid is:

　J'ai la paupière:

　　❑ red.

　　rouge.

　　❑ swollen.

　　enflée.

　　❑ painful.

　　douloureuse.

❑ I have no pain.

　Je n'ai pas mal.

❑ I have pain. (Refer to Visual Pain Scale)

　J'ai mal. (Voir echelle de douleur)

❑ The pain is:

　La douleur est:

　　❑ throbbing.

　　lancinante.

　　❑ dull.

　　sourde.

　　❑ sharp.

　　aiguë.

　　❑ intermittent.

　　intermittente.

　　❑ constant.

　　constante.

❑ The pain is located in the:

　La douleur est localisée dans:

❑ eye.
   l'œil.
❑ head.
   la tête.
❑ face.
   le visage.
❑ neck.
   la nuque.
❑ The pain does not radiate (move).
La douleur ne se propage pas (bouger).
❑ The pain radiates to my:
La douleur se propage:
   ❑ head.
      à la tête.
   ❑ face.
      au visage.
   ❑ neck.
      à la nuque.
❑ I have been exposed to:
J'ai été en contact avec:
   ❑ bright sunlight (skiing and water sports).
      un soleil très fort (au ski ou à la mer).
   ❑ welding.
      des éclats de soudure.
   ❑ chemicals.
      des produits chimiques.
   ❑ fumes.
      des fumées toxiques.
   ❑ infection.
      une infection.
❑ I am nauseated. (Refer to Nausea Section)
J'ai la nausée. (Voir section nausée)
❑ I have a fever. (Refer to Fever Section)
J'ai de la fièvre. (Voir section fièvre)
❑ I have a headache. (Refer to Headache Section)
J'ai mal à la tête. (Voir section mal à la tête)

❏ I have a toothache.

J'ai mal aux dents.

❏ I have ear pain or ringing.

J'ai une douleur ou une sonnerie dans l'oreille.

❏ I have used eye drops.

J'ai pris des gouttes pour les oreilles.

❏ I have taken medications. (Show medications)

J'ai pris des médicaments. (Montrer les médicaments)

❏ This has never happened before.

Cela ne m'est jamais arrivé.

❏ This has happened before ＿＿＿ days/years ago.

Cela m'est déjà arrivé, il y a ＿＿＿ jours/ans.

❏ I have no prior eye problems.

Je n'ai jamais eu de problèmes à l'œil.

❏ I wear glasses.

Je porte des lunettes.

❏ I wear contact lenses.

Je porte des lentilles de contact.

❏ I have:

J'ai:

   ❏ cataracts.

    une cataracte.

   ❏ glaucoma.

    un glaucome.

❏ I use medications for my eyes. (Refer to Medication Section)

Je prends des médicaments pour les yeux. (Voir section médicaments)

Pink Eye (Conjunctivitis)

Pink eye is a common malady that may require antibiotics to cure. The following section will assist you during an interview for pink eye. Pertinent information which will assist your physician is included in this section.

La conjonctivite

La conjonctivite est une maladie courante qui peut nécessiter des antibiotiques pour être soignée. La section ci-dessous vous aidera durant une consultation pour une conjonctivite. Cette section contient des informations importantes qui aideront votre médecin.

Check only those questions to which you answer YES.
Cochez seulement les questions auxquelles vous répondez OUI.

Complaint
Symptômes

❏ I have pink eye in the left/right/both eyes.
 J'ai une conjonctivite à l'œil droit/gauche/aux deux yeux.
❏ I have had this problem for _____ hours/days.
 J'ai ce problème depuis _____ heures/jours.
❏ I have pain in the affected eye(s).
 J'ai mal à l'œil/aux yeux affecté(s).
❏ I have diminished vision in my affected eye(s).
 Je vois moins bien de l'œil/des yeux affecté(s).
❏ I have blurred vision in my affected eye(s).
 Je vois flou de l'œil/des yeux affecté(s).
❏ I have double vision in my affected eye(s).
 Je vois double de l'œil/des yeux affecté(s).
❏ I cannot see out of my affected eye(s).
 Je ne vois rien de l'œil/des yeux affecté(s).

Associated symptoms and history
Symptômes associés et informations complémentaires

❏ I have some liquid draining from my affected eye(s).
 J'ai du liquide qui coule de l'œil/des yeux affecté(s).
❏ I have itchy eye(s).
 J'ai l'œil/les yeux qui me pique(nt).
❏ I have had no trauma to my eye(s).
 Je ne me suis pas fait mal à l'œil/aux yeux.
❏ I have something in my eye(s).
 J'ai quelque chose dans l'œil.
❏ I have a headache.
 J'ai mal à la tête.
❏ I wear contact lenses. They are hard/soft lenses.

Je porte des lentilles de contact. Ce sont des lentilles
rigides/souples.

❏ I have been wearing my contact lenses recently.
J'ai porté mes lentilles de contact récemment.

❏ I took my contact lenses out _____ minutes/hours/days ago.
J'ai enlevé mes lentilles de contact il y a _____ minutes/
heures/jours.

❏ I wear glasses.
Je porte des lunetttes.

❏ I feel like something is under my eyelid.
J'ai l'impression d'avoir quelque chose sous la paupière.

❏ I feel like something was blown into my eye(s).
J'ai l'impression d'avoir une poussière dans l'œil.

❏ I have not had any chemicals splashed into my eye(s).
Je n'ai pas reçu de produit chimique dans l'œil.

❏ I have had a chemical splashed into my eye(s).
J'ai reçu du produit chimique dans l'œil.

❏ The chemical exposure occurred _____ minutes/hours/days ago.
J'ai été en contact avec ce produit chimique il y a _____
minutes/heures/jours.

❏ The chemical was:
Il s'agissait:

  ❏ a household cleaner.
  d'un produit d'entretien ménager.

  ❏ a chemical from my car.
  d'un produit chimique provenant de ma voiture.

  ❏ a chemical from work.
  d'un produit chimique provenant de mon travail.

❏ I have been waking up with a thick substance coming from the
affected eye(s).
Lorsque je me réveille, j'ai une substance épaisse qui coule de
l'œil/des yeux affecté(s).

❏ I have had a hard time opening my eyes in the morning.
J'ai du mal à ouvrir les yeux le matin.

❏ Sometimes, my eyelids feel like they are stuck together in the morning.

Quelquefois, j'ai l'impression d'avoir les paupières collées le matin.

❏ I have glaucoma.

J'ai un glaucome.

❏ Please look at the rest of my medical history.

(Refer to Medical History Section)

Veuillez consulter le reste de la page concernant mes antécédents médicaux. (Voir antécédents médicaux)

❏ I have tried washing out my eye(s).

J'ai essayé de me rincer l'œil/les yeux.

❏ I have taken out my contact lenses.

J'ai enlevé mes lentilles de contact.

❏ I used some eye drops. These are the eye drops.

J'ai pris des gouttes pour les yeux. Les voici.

Nosebleed

Nose bleeding may be spontaneous or associated with systemic diseases such as hypertension. The assessment of nosebleeds is based upon identification of the location of the bleeding and evaluation of underlying aggravating diseases such as hypertension, bleeding disorders, etc. Local control by placement of gauze pads or "pledgets" soaked in a substance which causes blood vessels to contract is common. Different substances can be used to control the local blood flow (called vasoconstrictors) including cocaine, etc. Make sure that you inform the physician of any medical problem, allergies, and medications you are taking (both prescription and over the counter). Trauma may also be part of the history of nosebleeds. Although nosebleeds may seem trivial, treatment of other underlying medical problems is important for good outcome.

Treatment may include cauterization of the area with a silver nitrate stick, balloon tamponade, or a nose pack. Elderly patients may require hospitalization. Follow-up may include referral to an ear, nose, and throat specialist for further treatment.

Les saignements de nez

Les saignements de nez peuvent être spontanés ou bien liés à des maladies de l'organisme telles que l'hypertension. Le diagnostic des saignements de nez consiste à identifier la localisation du saignement; et à évaluer les facteurs aggravants tels que l'hypertension, les saignements anormaux, etc. Il est courant de remédier au saignement ponctuel en plaçant des bande de gaze ou des compresses imbibées d'une substance qui fait que les vaisseaux sanguins se contractent. Différentes substances peuvent être utilisées pour remédier à l'écoulement de sang ponctuel (on les appelle des vasoconstricteurs), y compris la cocaïne, etc. Veillez à bien informer le médecin de vos problèmes médicaux, de vos allergies et des médicaments que vous prenez (sur ordonnance et par auto-médication). Un traumatisme peut aussi partiellement expliquer des saignements de nez chroniques. Bien que les saignements de nez puissent sembler bénins, il est important de traiter les problèmes potentiels sous-jacents pour un résultat optimal.

Le traitement peut nécessiter une cautérisation de la zone affectée à l'aide d'une tige en nitrate d'argent, d'un méchage nasal, ou d'une compresse pour le nez. Il se peut que les patients âgés nécessitent une hospitalisation. Le suivi médical pourra inclure une consultation chez un ophtalmologiste ou un oto-rhino-laryngologiste pour un traitement approfondi.

Check only those questions to which you answer YES.
Cochez seulement les questions auxquelles vous répondez OUI.

Complaint
Symptômes
❏ I am bleeding from the (right/left/both) side(s) of my nose.
  Je saigne du côté droit/gauche/des deux côtés du nez.
❏ It has been bleeding for _____ hours/days.
  Je saigne du nez depuis _____ heures/jours.

Associated symptoms and history
Symptômes associés et informations complémentaires
❏ The bleeding started spontaneously.

Je me suis mis(e) à saigner du nez soudainement.

❏ There was no injury.

Je n'ai pas de blessure.

❏ There was an injury to my nose. (Demonstrate injury)

J'ai une blessure au nez. (Démontrer blessure)

❏ This has happened before.

Cela m'est déjà arrivé.

❏ I have frequent nosebleeds.

Je saigne souvent du nez.

❏ This has never happened before.

Cela ne m'est jamais arrivé.

❏ I have bleeding problems; I bleed easily.

J'ai des problèmes de saignement; Je saigne facilement.

❏ I do not have any known bleeding problems.

Je n'ai pas de problèmes de saignement identifiés.

❏ I am dizzy or lightheaded.

J'ai des vertiges ou j'ai la tête qui tourne.

❏ I am nauseated.

J'ai la nausée.

❏ I have put a packing/tissue in my nose.

Je me suis mis une compresse/un tampon dans le nez.

❏ I have compressed it for _____ minutes/hours.

Je l'ai comprimé pendant _____ minutes/heures.

❏ I have placed ice on it.

J'ai mis de la glace dessus.

Sinusitis and Colds

Most upper respiratory infections are caused by viruses and will resolve by themselves. Very few require antibiotics. Americans are more likely to be given antibiotics for upper respiratory infections by their doctors than people in other countries. The main goal is to relieve your symptoms and congestion.

Sinuses are cavities in your nose and in areas of your face and forehead that are connected to your nose. If these become filled with mucous and do not drain you may experience severe pain.

The doctor may prescribe pain medications, decongestants

(tablets or sprays), and possibly antibiotics. In many countries you will not be given antibiotics for these conditions. They are not incorrect in treating you this way. Most of these medications are available in a pharmacy without a prescription.

In some foreign countries you may be able to discuss this problem with a pharmacist. Review the over-the-counter medications that you use while in the United States. The trade name (such as Robitussin DM) will have the generic names below each listing. Select a medication which you would use and show the physician or pharmacist the name of it. This will assist in the selection of a similar medication.

Les sinusites et les rhumes

La plupart des infections respiratoires supérieures sont dues à des virus et se résolvent d'elles-mêmes. Très peu d'entre elles nécessitent des antibiotiques. Les médecins américains ont davantage tendance à donner des antibiotiques pour traiter les infections respiratoires supérieures que les médecins des autres pays. Les traitements principaux visent à soulager vos symptômes et votre congestion.

Les sinus sont des cavités situées dans le visage, le nez et le front, et reliées au nez. S'ils se remplissent de mucus et ne se débouchent pas, cela peut faire très mal.

Le docteur peut prescrire des antalgiques, des décongestionnants (comprimés ou pulvérisations) et éventuellement des antibiotiques. Gardez à l'esprit que dans beaucoup de pays, on ne vous donnera pas d'antibiotiques pour traiter ce problème. Les médecins de ces pays ne font pas d'erreurs en traitant le problème de la sorte. La plupart des médicaments pour les sinus sont vendus en pharmacie sans ordonnance.

Dans certains pays étrangers, il est possible que vous puissiez parler de ce problème avec un pharmacien. Consultez les médicaments américains que vous acheteriez en pharmacie pour votre consommation aux Etats-Unis. La marque de ce produit (Robitussin DM, par exemple) comprendra, au bas de la notice, la liste des noms génériques du produit. Choisissez le médicament que vous utiliseriez et montrez-le au médecin ou au pharmacien. Cela l'aidera à choisir un médicament similaire.

Check only those questions to which you answer YES.
Cochez seulement les questions auxquelles vous répondez OUI.

Complaint
Symptômes

❏ I have a problem with my sinuses. (Refer to Head Diagrams)
  J'ai un problème aux sinus. (Voir les diagrammes de la tête)
❏ I have a fever. (Refer to Temperature Scale)
  J'ai de la fièvre. (Voir l'échelle de température)
❏ I do not have drainage from my nose.
  Je n'ai pas d'écoulement du nez.
❏ I have drainage from my nose.
  J'ai un écoulement du nez.
❏ Its color is:
  Cet écoulement est:
    ❏ clear.
      clair.
    ❏ white.
      blanc.
    ❏ yellow.
      jaune.
    ❏ green.
      vert.
    ❏ bloody.
      contient du sang.
❏ This problem started _____ minutes/hours/days ago.
  Ce problème a débuté il y a _____ minutes/heures/jours.

Associated symptoms and history
Symptômes associés et informations complémentaires

❏ I have pain. (Refer to Visual Pain Scale)
  J'ai mal. (Voir l'échelle de douleur)
❏ The pain is:
  La douleur est:
    ❏ throbbing.
      lancinante.

❏ dull.

  sourde.

❏ sharp.

  aiguë.

❏ intermittent.

  intermittente.

❏ constant.

  constante.

❏ I have a cold.

  J'ai le rhume.

❏ I have ear pain.

  J'ai mal à l'oreille.

❏ I have a headache.

  J'ai mal à la tête.

❏ I have a toothache.

  J'ai mal aux dents.

❏ I am nauseated.

  J'ai la nausée.

❏ I have been swimming.

  Je me suis baigné(e).

❏ I have been underwater diving (scuba or snorkeling).

  J'ai fait de la plongée sous-marine (plongée bouteille ou masque et tuba).

❏ I have been traveling on airplanes.

  J'ai voyagé par avion.

❏ I have been in the mountains.

  Je suis allé(e) en montagne.

❏ I have used nose sprays.

  J'ai utilisé un vaporisateur nasal.

❏ I have taken medications.

  J'ai pris des médicaments.

❏ This has never happened before.

  Cela ne m'est jamais arrivé.

❏ This happened ____ days/months/years ago.

  Cela m'est arrivé il y a ____ jours/mais/ans.

❏ I have this happen frequently.

Cela m'arrive fréquemment.

❏ I have no prior sinus problems.

Je n'ai jamais eu de problèmes de sinus.

Sore Throat

Sore throat is an extremely common problem which sometimes requires medical attention. The following section will assist you in giving your healthcare provider pertinent information regarding a sore throat.

Les maux de gorge

Le mal de gorge est un problème extrêmement fréquent qui nécessite parfois des soins médicaux. La section ci-dessous vous aidera à fournir à votre praticien de santé des renseignements importants concernant votre mal de gorge.

Check only those questions to which you answer YES.
Cochez seulement les questions auxquelles vous répondez OUI.

Complaint
Symptômes

❏ I have a sore throat.

J'ai mal à la gorge.

❏ I have had this problem for _____ hours/days.

J'ai ce problème depuis _____ heures/jours.

❏ I have a fever of _____ degrees Fahrenheit/Celsius. (Refer to Temperature Scale)

J'ai de la fièvre. J'ai _____ Fahrenheit/Celsius de température. (Voir l'échelle de température)

❏ I have been vomiting. (Refer to Vomiting Section)

J'ai des vomissements. (Voir section vomissements)

Associated symptoms and history
Symptômes associés et informations complémentaires

❏ I have pain in my throat.

J'ai mal à la gorge.

❏ I am able to swallow fluids.

J'arrive à avaler des fluides.

❏ I have pain when I swallow.

J'ai mal quand j'avale.

❏ I am hoarse.

Je suis enroué(e).

❏ I have been hoarse for _____ hours/days.

Je suis enroué(e) depuis _____ heures/jours.

❏ I am having trouble breathing.

J'ai du mal à respirer.

❏ I have been drooling.

Je bave.

❏ I have pain in my sinuses. (Refer to Head Diagrams)

J'ai mal aux sinus. (Voir les diagrammes de la tête)

❏ I have a cough.

Je tousse.

❏ I have a rash.

J'ai de l'urticaire.

❏ I have a headache. (Refer to Headache Section)

J'ai mal à la tête. (Voir section mal à la tête)

❏ I have aches and pains in my muscles/joints/both.

J'ai des courbatures et des douleurs dans les muscles/les
articulations/les deux.

❏ Other members of my party are also sick.

D'autres personnes de mon groupe sont également malades.

❏ I smoke cigarettes. I smoke _____ cigarettes per day.

Je fume la cigarette. Je fume _____ cigarettes par jour.

❏ Please look at my other medical information.

Veuillez consulter les autres renseignements médicaux me
concernant.

Neck Pain

Neck pain may be the result of trauma or chronic inflammation of the
vertebral bodies of the cervical spine. The following will assist you in
providing pertinent information to your physician regarding this complaint.

Les douleurs dans la nuque

Les douleurs dans la nuque peuvent être la conséquence d'un traumatisme ou d'une inflammation chronique des vertébres cervicales. La section ci-dessous vous aidera à fournir à votre médecin des renseignements importants concernant cette douleur.

Check only those questions to which you answer YES.
Cochez seulement les questions auxquelles vous répondez OUI.

Complaint
Symptômes

❑ I have pain in my neck.
   J'ai mal à la nuque.
❑ I have pain in the right/left side.
   J'ai mal au côté droit/gauche.
❑ The pain has been present for _____ minutes/hours/days.
   J'ai cette douleur depuis _____ minutes/heures/jours.

Associated symptoms and history
Symptômes associés et informations complémentaires

❑ I have had a recent neck injury. This injury occurred
   _____ minutes/hours/days ago.
   Je me suis récemment fait mal à la nuque. C'était il y a
   _____ minutes/heures/jours.
❑ The pain is worse when I move right/left/back/forward.
   La douleur s'accentue quand je bouge la tête à droite/à gauche/en avant/en arrière.
❑ My recent injury was:
   Je me suis fait mal récemment:
   ❑ a fall.
      en tombant.
   ❑ an auto accident.
      dans un accident de voiture.
   ❑ a blow to the head.
      en me cognant la tête.
❑ My neck feels stiff.

J'ai une raideur dans la nuque.

❏ I have pain from my neck which goes into my right/left arm.

J'ai une douleur dans le cou qui se propage dans le bras
droit/gauche.

❏ I have a fever. (Refer to Temperature Scale)

J'ai de la fièvre. (Voir l'échelle de temperature)

❏ I have a sore throat.

J'ai mal à la gorge.

❏ I have a cold.

J'ai le rhume.

❏ I have nausea.

J'ai la nausée.

❏ I have been vomiting.

J'ai des vomissements.

❏ I have put a hot/cold compress on my neck.

Je me suis appliqué une compresse chaude/froide sur la nuque.

❏ I have taken pain medications. These are the pain medications.

J'ai pris des médicaments. Voici ces médicaments.

❏ I have rested my neck.

Je me suis reposé la nuque.

General Chest Complaints

Review this section if you are experiencing shortness of breath, cough
or chest discomfort. This section includes both chest pain associated
with cardiac (heart) problems and other complaints pertaining to the
pulmonary (lung) system. If you know that you are having heart related problems, you may wish to go to the section on cardiac diseases.
If you are unsure as to what the problem is it would be best to complete the following section. The section is comprehensive and should
be completed in its entirety.

Please be sure that the first section regarding your medical history, current medications, allergies, etc. has been filled out completely.

Les douleurs de poitrine générales

Consultez cette section si vous êtes essoufflé(e), si vous toussez, ou
si vous avez mal dans la poitrine. Cette section comprend à la fois les
douleurs de poitrine liées à des problèmes cardiaques et d'autres

douleurs appartenant au système pulmonaire. Si vous savez que vous avez des problèmes d'ordre cardiaque, il serait bon de consulter la section sur les maladies cardiaques. Cette section est exhaustive et doit être complétée dans sa totalité.

Veuillez vous assurer d'avoir complété soigneusement la section I concernant vos antécédents médicaux, vos traitements en cours, et vos allergies, etc.

Check only those questions to which you answer YES.
Cochez seulement les questions auxquelles vous répondez OUI.

Complaint
Symptômes
❑ I have shortness of breath. The shortness of breath came on:
   Je suis essoufflé(e). Cet essoufflement est survenu:
   ❑ slowly.
      lentement.
   ❑ all of a sudden.
      tout à coup.
❑ I have chest pain. The chest pain came on:
   J'ai une douleur à la poitrine. Cette douleur est survenue:
   ❑ slowly.
      lentement.
   ❑ all of a sudden.
      tout à coup.
❑ The problem started _____ minutes/hours/days ago.
   Le problème a débuté il y a _____ minutes/heures/jours.
❑ I have a fever, chills, and sweats. (Refer to Temperature Scale)
   J'ai de la fièvre, des frissons et des suées. (Voir l'échelle de temperature)

Associated symptoms and history
Symptômes associés et informations complémentaires
❑ The shortness of breath is worse when I lie down.
   Je suis encore plus essoufflé(e) quand je m'étends.
❑ I have woken from sleep because I was short of breath.
   Je me suis réveillé(e) parce que j'étais essoufflé(e).

❏ I sleep in a chair.
  Je dors dans un fauteuil.
❏ I have wheezing.
  J'ai une respiration sifflante.
❏ I have noticed that my ankles are getting larger.
  J'ai constaté que mes chevilles avaient gonflé.
❏ I have a cough.
  Je tousse.
❏ I have felt well up until this problem started.
  Je me sentais bien avant d'avoir ce problème.
❏ I am in good health.
  Je suis en bonne santé.
❏ I have medical problems. (Refer to Medical History Section)
  J'ai des problèmes de santé. (Voir antécédents médicaux)
❏ I feel like I cannot catch my breath.
  J'ai l'impression de ne pas arriver à reprendre mon souffle.
❏ I have chest pain here: (Refer to Chest Diagrams)
  J'ai une douleur à la poitrine à cet endroit-là : insérer le diagramme
    de la poitrine. (Voir les diagrammes de la poitrine)
❏ When I take a deep breath, I have chest pain here:
    (Refer to Chest Diagrams)
  Quand j'inspire profondément, j'ai une douleur à la poitrine à cet
    endroit-là: (Voir les diagrammes de la poitrine)
❏ I have chest pain when I cough or sneeze.
  J'ai une douleur à la poitrine quand je tousse ou éternue.
❏ The pain is relieved when I press against this area with my hand.
  La douleur s'atténue quand j'appuie sur cet endroit-là avec
    ma main.
❏ I have asthma.
  J'ai de l'asthme.
❏ I have asthma which has required hospitalization in the past.
  J'ai déjà dû être hospitalisé(e) à cause de mon asthme.
❏ I have lung problems which have required steroid therapy in the
    past.
  J'ai déjà dû prendre des stéroïdes à cause de mes problèmes de
    poumon.

❏ I have a cough.
  Je tousse.
❏ My cough produces sputum which is:
  Quand je tousse, je crache une substance qui est:
    ❏ clear.
      clair.
    ❏ yellow.
      jaune.
    ❏ green.
      verte.
    ❏ reddish (like rust).
      rougeâtre (comme de la rouille).
    ❏ putrid smelling.
      qui sent le pourri.
❏ I have had pain in my right/left leg.
  J'ai déjà eu mal à la jambe droite/gauche.
❏ My right/left leg has been swollen.
  Ma jambe droite/gauche a déjà été enflée.
❏ I have been sitting for a long period of time.
  Je suis resté longtemps assis.
❏ I have been drinking alcohol.
  J'ai bu de l'alcool.
❏ I passed out before my chest pain began.
  Je me suis évanoui(e) avant que cette douleur à la poitrine ne
  débute.
❏ I passed out after I coughed very heavily.
  Je me suis évanoui(e) après avoir toussé très violemment.
❏ I have a rash.
  J'ai de l'urticaire.
❏ I have oral ulcers.
  J'ai des ulcères à la bouche.
❏ I have bone pain.
  J'ai mal dans les os.
❏ I have been coughing up blood.
  Je crache du sang.
❏ The amount of blood which I have coughed up is:

La quantité de sang que j'ai crachée correspond à:
❏ several teaspoons.
   plusieurs cuillerées à café.
❏ several tablespoons.
   plusieurs cuillerées à soupe.
❏ less than a half cup.
   moins de _____ dls.
❏ I don't know.
   je ne sais pas.
❏ I feel like I may have pneumonia.
   On dirait que j'ai une pneumonie.
❏ I smoke cigarettes.
   Je fume des cigarettes.
❏ I smoke _____ packs of cigarettes per day.
   Je fume _____ paquets de cigarettes par jour.
❏ I smoke _____ cigars per day.
   Je fume _____ cigares par jour.
❏ I smoke a pipe.
   Je fume la pipe.
❏ I have smoked for _____ years.
   Je fume depuis _____ ans.
❏ I have emphysema.
   J'ai de l'emphysème.
❏ I have had tuberculosis.
   J'ai eu la tuberculose.
❏ I have bronchitis.
   J'ai une bronchite.
❏ I have bronchiectasis.
   J'ai une bronchiectasie.
❏ I have abdominal pain in addition to my shortness of breath.
   (Refer to Abdominal Pain Section)
   J'ai une douleur abdominale en plus d'être essoufflé(e).
   (Voir section douleur abdominale)
❏ The chest pain is present but is not made worse or better by
   breathing.
   Cette douleur à la poitrine est présente mais le fait d'inspirer ou

d'expirer ne me fait ni plus mal ni moins mal.

❑ The chest pain is under my left breast.
Cette douleur à la poitrine se situe sous mon sein gauche.

❑ The chest pain gets worse when I walk. I can only walk _____
blocks before I have to stop.
Cette douleur à la poitrine s'accentue quand je marche. Je ne peux
parcourir à pied que la distance entre _____ rues avant de
m'arrêter.

❑ The chest pain starts in my chest and radiates to my neck.
Cette douleur à la poitrine commence dans la poitrine et se
propage dans la nuque.

❑ I have pain in my right/left/both arm(s).
J'ai mal au bras droit/gauche/aux deux.

❑ I have pain in my right/left/both hand(s).
J'ai mal à la main droit/gauche/aux deux.

❑ My left hand feels numb.
Je n'ai plus de sensation dans la main gauche.

❑ The chest pain feels like a crushing sensation under my chest bone.
(Refer to Chest Diagrams)
Quand je ressens cette douleur à la poitrine, c'est comme si on me
broyait la cage thoracique.
(Voir les diagrammes de la poitrine)

❑ The chest pain is a dull aching sensation.
Cette douleur à la poitrine est une douleur sourde.

❑ The chest pain began when I was emotionally distressed.
Cette douleur à la poitrine a commencé après une forte émotion.

❑ The chest pain usually lasts several minutes.
Cette douleur à la poitrine dure généralement quelques minutes.

❑ The chest pain began when I was outside in the cold air.
Cette douleur à la poitrine a commencé alors que je me trouvais
dehors au froid.

❑ The chest pain began after I ate a meal.
J'ai commencé à ressentir cette douleur à la poitrine après avoir
mangé.

❑ The chest pain woke me from a sound sleep at _____ o'clock
AM/PM.

Cette douleur à la poitrine m'a réveillé(e) alors que je dormais
profondément à _____ heures du matin/de l'après-midi/du soir.

❑ The chest pain came on while I was at rest.
Cette douleur à la poitrine est survenue alors que je me reposais.

❑ The chest pain is sharp and starts under my left breast.
Cette douleur à la poitrine est aiguë et commence sous mon sein
gauche.

❑ The chest pain radiates to: (Refer to Chest Diagrams)
(This question is directed at pericarditis and possible radiation.)
Cette douleur dans la poitrine se propage à/au: (Voir les
diagrammes de la poitrine)
(La question est liée aux péricardites et à de possibles irradiations.)

❑ I have a tender spot here. (This is for costochondritis.)
Cet endroit-ci est sensible. (Ceci concerne les costochondrites)

❑ I have recently injured my chest. The injury occurred here.
(Refer to Chest Diagrams)
Je me suis récemment fait mal à la poitrine. Je me suis fait mal à
cet endroit-là. (Voir les diagrammes de la poitrine)

❑ I have neck pain. The pain is here. (Refer to Neck Diagrams)
J'ai mal dans le cou/la nuque. J'ai mal là. (Voir les diagrammes
du cou)

❑ The neck pain starts in my neck and radiates into my left arm and
shoulder.
Cette douleur dans la nuque commence dans la nuque et se propage
dans le bras gauche et dans l'épaule.

❑ The pain in my left arm is a chronic aching sensation.
La douleur que je ressens dans le bras gauche s'apparente à une
courbature chronique.

❑ I also sometimes feel like my hand is numb.
J'ai parfois l'impression de ne plus avoir de sensations dans la
main.

❑ My arm(s) is/are weak. The right/left is weaker than the other arm.
Mon bras est/Mes bras sont mou(s). Le droit/le gauche est plus
mou que l'autre bras.

❑ The arm pain is worse when I move my neck.
Cette douleur dans le bras s'accentue quand je bouge la nuque.

❏ The arm pain is worse when I raise my arm(s).
Cette douleur dans le bras s'accentue quand je lève le bras.

❏ I have been very anxious lately.
Je suis angoissé(e) depuis quelque temps.

❏ The chest pain is my usual angina pain. It has not changed.
Cette douleur à la poitrine correspond à mon angine de poitrine habituelle. Elle n'a pas changé.

❏ The chest pain is my usual angina pain. It has become worse. It is:
Cette douleur à la poitrine correspond à mon angine de poitrine habituelle. Mais elle s'est accentuée. Elle est:

  ❏ more/less frequent.
  plus/moins fréquente.

  ❏ more/less intense.
  plus/moins intense.

  ❏ of longer duration.
  dure plus longtemps.

❏ I have been having an irregular heartbeat (palpitations). It feels like:
J'ai le cœur qui bat irrégulièrement (j'ai des palpitations). Cela fait comme:

  ❏ a pounding or thumping in my chest.
  un bruit sourd et fort dans ma poitrine.

  ❏ a rapid flutter in my chest.
  un battement rapide dans ma poitrine.

❏ I nearly passed out when I started having chest pain.
Je me suis presque évanoui(e) quand j'ai commencé à ressentir cette douleur à la poitrine.

❏ I passed out when I started having chest pain.
Je me suis évanoui(e) quand j'ai commencé à ressentir cette douleur à la poitrine.

❏ I have a history of seizures.
Je fais très souvent des crises.

❏ I have never had a history of seizures.
Je n'ai jamais eu de crises à répétition.

❏ I lost control of my bowels when I passed out.
J'ai déféqué sans m'en rendre compte quand je me suis évanoui(e).

❑ I lost control of my urine when I passed out.

J'ai uriné sans m'en rendre compte quand je me suis évanoui(e).

❑ I sweat when I have chest pain.

J'ai des suées quand je ressens cette douleur à la poitrine.

❑ I have nausea when I have chest pain.

J'ai des nausées quand je ressens cette douleur à la poitrine.

❑ I have vomited when I have had chest pain.

Je vomis quand je ressens cette douleur à la poitrine.

Medical History
Antécédents Médicaux

❑ I have high blood pressure.

J'ai une tension artérielle élevée.

❑ I have high cholesterol.

J'ai un taux de cholestérol élevé.

❑ I have high lipids.

J'ai un taux de lipides élevé.

❑ I have a family history of:

Dans ma famille, il y a beaucoup de:

  ❑ heart disease.

    maladies cardiaques.

  ❑ high blood pressure.

    problèmes de tension artérielle élevée.

  ❑ high cholesterol.

    problèmes de taux de cholestérol élevé.

  ❑ myocardial infarct in a close relative under the age of 50.

    d'infarctus du myocarde dans ma famille proche avant l'âge de 50 ans.

  ❑ I have tuberculosis.

    J'ai la tuberculose.

  ❑ I have Systemic Lupus Erythematosis (SLE).

    J'ai un Lupus Erythémateux Aigu Disséminé.

  ❑ I have Rheumatoid Arthritis.

    J'ai de l'arthrite rhumatoïde.

  ❑ I have sarcoidosis.

    J'ai une sarcoïdose.

Cough

This section is designed to report the information regarding cough. Cough may be acute or chronic. Some coughs may be associated with medications. Think carefully about the duration of your cough, precipitating factors, and any history associated with lung disease, especially smoking.

La toux

Cette section a été conçue pour fournir des renseignements concernant la toux. La toux peut apparaître soudainement ou être chronique. Certaines toux peuvent être liées à une prise de médicaments. Réfléchissez bien à la durée de votre toux, aux facteurs qui ont pu hâter son développement, et à tout antécédent médical lié à une maladie des poumons, et particulièrement au fait de fumer.

Check only those questions to which you answer YES.
Cochez seulement les questions auxquelles vous répondez OUI.

Complaint
Symptômes
❑ I have a cough.
   Je tousse.
❑ The problem has been present for ____minutes/hours/days/weeks.
   J'ai ce problème depuis _____ minutes/heures/jours/semaines.

Associated symptoms and history
Symptômes associés et informations complémentaires
❑ I have had aches and pains in my muscles and my joints.
   J'ai des courbatures et des douleurs dans les muscles et les
      articulations.
❑ I have a fever. (Refer to Temperature Scale)
   J'ai de fièvre. (Voir l'échelle de température)
❑ I have had to sleep in an upright position.
   J'ai dû dormir à-demi allongé(e).
❑ I have post-nasal drip.
   J'ai un écoulement post-nasal.
❑ I have sinusitis. (Refer to Head Diagrams)
   J'ai une sinusite. (Voir les diagrammes de la tête)

❏ When I cough, I produce:
  Quand je tousse, je crache:
   ❏ blood.
     du sang.
   ❏ white sputum.
     une substance blanche.
   ❏ rust colored sputum.
     une substance de la couleur de la rouille.
   ❏ yellow sputum.
     une substance jaune.
   ❏ green sputum.
     une substance verte.
❏ I have asthma.
  J'ai de l'asthme.
❏ I am short of breath.
  Je suis essoufflé(e).
❏ I have wheezing.
  J'ai une respiration sifflante.
❏ I smoke _____ packs of cigarettes per day.
  Je fume _____ paquets de cigarettes par jour.
❏ I smoke _____ cigars per day.
  Je fume _____ cigares par jour.
❏ I smoke a pipe.
  Je fume la pipe.
❏ I have smoked for _____ years.
  Je fume depuis _____ ans.
❏ I have been treated with steroids (prednisone) in the past for this
    problem.
  J'ai déjà été traité(e) avec des stéroïdes (prednisone) pour ce
    problème.
❏ I have bronchitis.
  J'ai une bronchite.
❏ I have gastroesophageal reflux disease (GERD).
  J'ai un reflux gastro-œsophagien.
❏ I have bronchiectasis.
  J'ai une bronchiectasie.

❏ I have nasal congestion.
J'ai une congestion nasale.

❏ I have a runny nose.
J'ai le nez qui coule.

❏ I have a sore throat.
J'ai mal à la gorge.

❏ I have an earache in my right/left ear. (Refer to Ear Problems Section)
J'ai mal à l'oreille dans l'oreille droite/l'oreille gauche. (Voir section oreille)

❏ I have a pressure sensation in my head. (Refer to Head Diagrams)
J'ai une sensation de pression dans la tête. (Voir les diagrammes de la tête)

❏ I have chest pain when I take a deep breath.
J'ai mal à la poitrine quand j'inspire profondément.

❏ I have had swelling in both of my legs.
J'ai les deux jambes enflées.

❏ I have swelling and tenderness in my right/left leg. (Refer to Leg Diagrams)
J'ai la jambe droite/gauche qui est enflée et sensible. (Voir les diagrammes des jambes)

❏ I lost consciousness recently.
Je me suis évanoui(e) récemment.

❏ I have had a stiff neck.
J'ai une raideur dans la nuque.

Shortness of Breath

This section is designed to review the pertinent information regarding shortness of breath. If you are sure that your current problem is lung related, complete this section. If you are unsure as to what is causing your problem, please review the general Chest Section.

L'essoufflement

Cette section a été conçue pour passer en revue les informations importantes concernant l'essoufflement. Si vous êtes sûr(e) que votre problème actuel est lié au poumon, complétez cette section. Si vous n'êtes pas sûr(e) de la cause de votre problème, veuillez consulter la section générale sur la poitrine.

Check only those questions to which you answer YES.
Cochez seulement les questions auxquelles vous répondez OUI.

Complaint
Symptômes
❏ I have shortness of breath. The shortness of breath came on:
  Je suis essoufflé(e). Cet essoufflement est survenu:
    ❏ slowly.
      lentement.
    ❏ all of a sudden.
      soudainement.
❏ The problem began _____ minutes/hours/days/weeks ago.
  Ce problème a débuté il y a _____ minutes/heures/jours/semaines.

Associated symptoms and history
Symptômes associés et informations complémentaires
❏ The shortness of breath is worse when I lie down.
  Je suis plus essoufflé(e) quand je m'allonge.
❏ I have woken from sleep because I was short of breath.
  Je me suis réveillé(e) parce que j'étais essoufflé(e).
❏ I sleep upright in a chair.
  Je dors assis(e) dans un fauteuil.
❏ I have wheezing.
  J'ai une respiration sifflante.
❏ I have noticed that my ankles are getting larger.
  J'ai constaté que mes chevilles avaient gonflé.
❏ I have felt well up until this problem started.
  Je me sentais bien avant d'avoir ce problème.
❏ I am in good health.
  Je suis en bonne santé.
❏ I feel like I cannot catch my breath.
  J'ai l'impression de ne pas arriver à reprendre mon souffle.
❏ I have chest pain here: (Refer to Chest Diagrams)

J'ai mal à la poitrine à cet endroit-là: (Voir les diagrammes de la poitrine)

❏ When I take a deep breath, I have chest pain here: (Refer to Chest Diagrams)
Lorsque j'inspire profondément, j'ai mal à la poitrine à cet endroit-là: (Voir les diagrammes de la poitrine.)

❏ I have asthma.
J'ai de l'asthme.

❏ I have asthma which has required hospitalization in the past.
J'ai déjà été hospitalisé(e) à cause de mon asthme.

❏ I have lung problems which have required steroid therapy in the past.
On m'a déjà prescrit des stéroïdes pour des problèmes de poumon.

❏ I have a cough.
Je tousse.

❏ My cough produces sputum which is:
Quand je tousse, je crache une substance qui est:

    ❏ clear.
    clair.

    ❏ yellow.
    jaune.

    ❏ green.
    verte.

    ❏ reddish (like rust).
    rougeâtre (comme de la rouille).

    ❏ putrid smelling.
    qui sent le pourri.

❏ I have a fever, chills, and sweats. (Refer to Temperature Scale)
J'ai de la fièvre, de frissons et des suées. (Voir l'échelle de temperature)

❏ I smoke _____ packs of cigarettes per day.
Je fume _____ paquets de cigarettes par jour.

❏ I smoke _____ cigars per day.
Je fume _____ cigares par jour.

❏ I smoke a pipe.
Je fume la pipe.

❏ I have smoked for _____ years.
  Je ne fume plus depuis _____ ans.
❏ I do not smoke.
  Je ne fume pas.
❏ I have had pain in my right/left leg.
  J'ai mal à la jambe droite/gauche.
❏ My right/left leg has been swollen lately.
  Ma jambe droite/gauche est enflée depuis quelque temps.
❏ I have been sitting for a long period of time.
  J'ai été longtemps assis(e).
❏ My ankle swelling began after I was sitting for a long period of
  time.
  Ma cheville a commencé à gonfler après que j'ai été longtemps
  assis(e).
❏ I have been coughing up blood.
  Je crache du sang.
❏ I have had recent trauma to my chest. (Refer to Chest Diagrams)
  J'ai eu récemment un traumatisme à la poitrine. (Voir les
  diagrammes de la poitrine)
❏ The amount of blood which I have coughed up is:
  La quantité de sang que je crache correspond à:
    ❏ several teaspoons.
      plusieurs cuillerées à café.
    ❏ several tablespoons.
      plusieurs cuillerées à soupe.
    ❏ less than half a cup.
      moins de _____ dls.
    ❏ I don't know.
      Je ne sais pas.
❏ I feel like I may have pneumonia.
  J'ai l'impression d'avoir une pneumonie.
❏ I have abdominal pain in addition to my shortness of breath. (Refer
  to Abdominal Pain Section)
  J'ai des douleurs abdominales en plus d'être essoufflé(e). (Voir la
  section des douleurs abdominales)

Asthma

Asthma is a common condition that can be very aggressive at times. This section is designed for patients with a known history of asthma. If you have a cough or are short of breath, please thoroughly read through the questions in the Chest Section.

L'asthme

L'asthme est un phénomène courant qui peut parfois être très sérieux. Cette section concerne les patients qui ont fréquemment des crises d'asthme. Si vous toussez ou si vous êtes essoufflé(e), veuillez parcourir attentivement les questions de la section concernant la poitrine.

Check only the questions to which you answer YES.
Cochez seulement les questions auxquelles vous répondez OUI.

Complaint
Symptômes

❏ I have asthma.
  J'ai de l'asthme.
❏ I am having an asthma attack.
  Je suis en train d'avoir une crise d'asthme.
❏ The asthma attack has lasted for _____ hours.
  La crise d'asthme a duré pendant _____ heures.
❏ The asthma symptoms have been getting worse over the
  past _____ minutes/hours/days.
  Les symptômes de l'asthme se sont aggravés au cours
  des _____ derniers/dernières minutes/heures/jours.

Associated symptoms and history
Symptômes associés et informations complémentaires

❏ I am short of breath.
  Je suis essoufflé(e).
❏ I have chest tightness. (Refer to Chest Pain Section)
  J'ai une sensation d'oppression au niveau de la poitrine.
  (Voir la section concernant les douleurs de poitrine)
❏ I have a cough at night.
  Je tousse la nuit.

❑ I have a cough early in the morning.
  Je tousse tôt le matin.
❑ I have a fever. My temperature is _____Centigrade/Fahrenheit.
  (Refer to Temperature Scale)
  J'ai de la fièvre. Ma température est de _____
  Centigrades/Farenheit.
  (Voir l'échelle de température)
❑ My cough is productive.
  Je crache quand je tousse.
❑ I am coughing up blood.
  Je crache du sang.
❑ I smoke cigarettes. I smoke _____ packs per day.
  Je fume des cigarettes. Je fume _____ paquets par jour.
❑ I have been exposed to cold air.
  J'ai été exposé à de l'air froid.
❑ I have been exposed to air pollution.
  J'ai été exposé à de la pollution atmosphérique.
❑ I have been exposed to strong odors.
  J'ai été en contact avec de fortes odeurs.
❑ I have an upper respiratory tract infection.
  J'ai une infection des voies respiratoires supérieures.
❑ I have an aspirin sensitivity.
  Je supporte mal l'aspirine.
❑ I have a history of heart problems. (Show your Medical History)
  J'ai déjà eu des problèmes cardiaques. (Montrez vos antécédents
  médicaux)
❑ I have had to be placed on a respirator in the past.
  On a déjà dû me mettre sous respirateur.
❑ I have been treated with steroids in the past.
  On m'a déjà traité(e) aux stéroïdes.
❑ I take medications for maintenance therapy. (Refer to Medications
  Section)
  Je prends des médicaments pour une thérapie d'entretien. (Voir
  section concernant les médicaments)
❑ I have been taking these medications. (Show medications)

Je prends ces médicaments-ci. (Montrer les médicaments)
❑ I last took these medications _____. (Date and time)
J'ai pris ces médicaments pour la dernière fois
_____. (Indiquer la date et l'heure)
❑ I have chronic bronchitis.
J'ai une bronchite chronique.
❑ I have cystic fibrosis.
J'ai une fibrose kystique (mucoviscidose).

Heart

This section is specific for cardiac problems. If you are sure you are experiencing cardiac problems, you should review this section in detail. If you are unsure about the problem you are experiencing, you should review the questions in the General Chest Complaints Section, which covers both lung and cardiac diseases. Many diseases may cause chest pain. These include acute myocardial infarction (MI or heart attack) as well as inflammation of the tissues which surround the heart (pericarditis).

Review the questions below carefully prior to checking the boxes. Read the entire section and then fill out the sections as accurately as possible.

If you have a history of coronary artery disease, it is extremely important that you fill out the Medical History Section completely. Include all hospitalizations, angiograms (results and dates), exercise stress tests, etc. Be sure that your medications include doses and frequency and are up to date. If possible, medications that have been used in the past, but which you have discontinued either due to allergy or for lack of efficacy should be included.

Le cœur

Cette section concerne spécifiquement les problèmes cardiaques. Si vous êtes sûr(e) d'avoir des problèmes cardiaques, examinez en détail cette section. Si vous n'êtes pas sûr(e) de ce dont vous souffrez, consultez la section générale sur les douleurs de poitrine. La section générale sur les douleurs de poitrine passe en revue des questions très importantes concernant les maladies cardiaques et pulmonaires. De nombreuses maladies peuvent occasionner des douleurs de poitrine.

Ces maladies comprennent les graves infarctus du moycarde, (IM ou crises cardiaques) et les inflammations des tissus qui enveloppent le cœur (péricardites).

Considérer attentivment les questions ci-dessous avant de cocher la bonn réponse. Veuillez lire l'ensemble de la section avant de la compléter aussi précisément que possible.

Si vous souffrez d'une maladie chronique des artères coronaires, il est extrêmement important que vous complétiez soigneusement la section sur les antécédents médicaux. Faites-y figurer toutes vos hospitalisations, vos angiogrammes (résultats et dates), vos examens cardiaques de stress, etc. Assurez-vous que vos médicaments spécifient dosages et fréquence, et qu'ils ne sont pas périmés. Dans la mesure du possible, faites figurer les médicaments que vous avez déjà utilisés, mais que vous avez cessé de prendre en raison d'une allergie ou d'un manque d'efficacité.

Check only those questions to which you answer YES.
Cochez seulement les questions auxquelles vous répondez OUI.

Complaint
Symptômes
❏ I have chest pain. (Refer to Chest Diagrams)
  J'ai mal dans la poitrine. (Voir les diagrammes de la poitrine)
❏ This problem has been present for _____ minutes/hours/days.
  J'ai ce problème depuis _____ minutes/heures/jours.

Associated symptoms and history
Symptômes associés et informations complémentaires
❏ The chest pain is present but is not made worse or better by
  breathing.
  Cette douleur dans la poitrine est présente mais elle ne
  s'accentue pas, ni ne s'atténue, quand je respire profondément.
❏ The chest pain is under my right/left breast.
  Cette douleur dans la poitrine se situe sous le sein droite/gauche.
❏ The chest pain starts in my chest and radiates to my neck.
  (Demonstrate)
  La douleur débute dans la poitrine et se propage dans la nuque.
  (Démontrer)

❑ I have pain in my right/left arm.
  J'ai mal au bras droit/gauche.
❑ I have pain in my right/left hand.
  J'ai mal à la main droite/gauche.
❑ My right/left hand feels numb.
  J'ai l'impression que ma main droite/gauche est n'a plus de
  sensations.
❑ The chest pain feels like a crushing sensation under my chest bone.
  Quand je ressens cette douleur dans la poitrine, j'ai l'impression
  qu'on me broie la cage thoracique.
❑ The chest pain is a dull aching sensation.
  Cette douleur dans la poitrine est sourde.
❑ The chest pain began when I was emotionally distressed.
  Cette douleur dans la poitrine a commencé après une forte
  émotion.
❑ The chest pain usually lasts several minutes.
  Cette douleur dans la poitrine dure généralement quelques
  minutes.
❑ The chest pain began when I was outside in the cold air.
  Cette douleur dans la poitrine a commencé alors que je me
  trouvais dehors dans le froid.
❑ The chest pain began after I ate a meal.
  Cette douleur dans la poitrine a commencé après un repas.
❑ The chest pain woke me from a sound sleep at _____ AM/PM.
  Cette douleur dans la poitrine m'a réveillé(e) alors que je
  dormais profondément à _____ du matin.
❑ The chest pain has been present constantly since the time it began.
  Je ressens cette douleur dans la poitrine constamment depuis
  qu'elle a commencé.
❑ The chest pain is present when I exert myself.
  Cette douleur dans la poitrine est présente quand je fais des
  efforts importants.
❑ The chest pain came on while I was at rest.
  Cette douleur dans la poitrine est survenue alors que je me
  reposais.
❑ The chest pain is sharp and starts under my left breast.

Cette douleur dans la poitrine est aiguë et commence sous le sein gauche.

❏ The chest pain radiates to: (Refer to Chest Diagrams) This question is directed at pericarditis and possible radiation.
Cette douleur dans la poitrine se propage dans: (Voir les diagrammes de la poitrine.) Cette question concerne directement les péricardites et les possibles irradiations.

❏ I have a tender spot here: (Refer to Chest Diagrams) This is for costochondritis.
Cet endroit-ci est sensible (Voir les diagrammes de la poitrine.). Ceci concerne les costochondrites.

❏ I have recently injured my chest. The injury occurred here: (Refer to Chest Diagrams)
Je me suis récemment fait mal à la poitrine. Je me suis fait mal là: (Voir les diagrammes de la poitrine.)

❏ I have neck pain. The pain is here: (Refer to Neck Diagrams)
J'ai mal dans la nuque. J'ai mal là. (Voir les diagrammes du cou)

❏ The neck pain starts in my neck and radiates into my right/left arm and shoulder.

❏ La douleur dans la nuque commence dans la nuque et se propage dans le bras et l'épaule droit/gauches.

❏ The pain in my left arm is a chronic aching sensation. I also sometimes feel like my hand is numb.
La douleur dans le bras gauche s'apparente à une courbature chronique. J'ai aussi parfois l'impression que ma main est n'a plus de sensations.

❏ My arm(s) is/are weak. The right/left is weaker than the other arm.
Mon bras/mes bras est/sont mou(s). Le droit/gauche est plus mou que l'autre bras.

❏ The arm pain is worse when I move my neck. (Demonstrate)
La douleur dans le bras s'intensifie quand je bouge la nuque. (Démontrer)

❏ The arm pain is worse when I raise my arm(s). (Demonstrate)
La douleur dans le bras s'intensifie quand je lève le bras. (Démontrer)

❏ I have been very anxious lately.

Je suis très angoissé(e) depuis quelque temps.

❏ The chest pain is my usual angina pain. It has not changed.
Cette douleur dans la poitrine correspond à mon angine de
poitrine habituelle. Elle n'a pas changé.

❏ The chest pain is my usual angina pain but it has become worse.
It is:
Cette douleur dans la poitrine correspond à mon angine de
poitrine habituelle. Elle est:

   ❏ more frequent.
   plus fréquente.

   ❏ more intense.
   plus intense.

   ❏ of longer duration.
   elle dure plus longtemps.

❏ I have been having an irregular heartbeat (palpitations). It feels
like:
J'ai le cœur qui bat de façon irrégulière (j'ai des palpitations).
Cela fait comme:

   ❏ a pounding or thumping in my chest.
   un bruit sourd et fort dans la poitrine.

   ❏ a rapid flutter in my chest.
   un battement rapide dans la poitrine.

❏ I have a history of irregular heartbeats. (Please review the Medical
History Section.)
J'ai souvent le cœur qui bat de façon irrégulière. (Veuillez
consulter mes antécédents médicaux.)

❏ I have felt this sensation before. (Refer to Medical History Section)
J'ai déjà ressenti cette sensation. (Voir antécédents médicaux)

❏ I nearly passed out when I started having chest pain.
Je me suis presque évanoui(e) quand j'ai commencé à ressentir
cette douleur à la poitrine.

❏ I passed out when I started having chest pain.
Je me suis évanoui(e) quand j'ai commencé à ressentir cette
douleur à la poitrine.

❏ I have a history of seizures.
Je fais souvent des crises.

❏ I have never had a history of seizures.

Je n'ai jamais eu de crises à répétition.

❏ I lost control of my bowels when I passed out. (Refer to Seizure
Section)

J'ai déféqué sans m'en rendre compte quand je me suis évanoui(e).
(Voir section attaques cérébrales)

❏ I lost control of my urine when I passed out. (Refer to Seizure
Section)

J'ai uriné sans m'en rendre compte quand je me suis évanoui(e).
(Voir section attaques cérébrales)

❏ I sweat when I have chest pain.

J'ai des suées quand je ressens cette douleur à la poitrine.

❏ I have nausea when I have chest pain.

J'ai des nausées quand je ressens cette douleur à la poitrine.

❏ I vomited when I had the chest pain.

Je vomis quand je ressens cette douleur à la poitrine.

❏ I have high blood pressure.

J'ai une tension artérielle élevée.

❏ I have high cholesterol.

J'ai un taux élevé de cholestérol.

❏ I have high lipids.

J'ai un taux élevé de lipides.

❏ I have a family history of:

Dans ma famille, il y a beaucoup de:

    ❏ heart disease.

    maladies cardiaques.

    ❏ high blood pressure.

    problèmes de tension artérielle élevée.

    ❏ high cholesterol.

    problèmes de taux de cholestérol élevé.

    ❏ myocardial infarct in a close relative under the age of 50.

    d'infarctus du myocarde survenant chez un proche avant
      l'âge de 50 ans.

❏ I smoke cigarettes.

Je fume des cigarettes.

❏ I smoke _____ cigarettes per day.

Je fume _____ cigarettes par jour.

❏ I smoke cigars.

Je fume le cigare.

❏ I smoke _____ cigars per day.

Je fume _____ cigares par jour.

❏ I do not smoke.

Je ne fume pas.

❏ I have smoked for _____ years.

Je fume depuis _____ années.

❏ I have taken my usual medications. (Refer to Medications Section)

J'ai pris mes médicaments habituels. (Voir section médicaments)

❏ I have taken more nitroglycerin. I have taken _____ (number) tablets.

J'ai pris davantage de nitroglycérine. J'ai pris _____ (nombre) comprimés.

❏ I have tried antacids. These have not changed the pain.

J'ai essayé des antacides. Ils n'ont pas changé la douleur.

❏ I have tried antacids. These have improved the pain but not completely resolved the problem. (Refer to Abdominal Pain Section)

J'ai essayé des antacides. Ils ont soulagé la douleur, mais ils n'ont pas complètement résolu le problème. (Voir la section des douleurs abdominales)

Abdominal Pain

Abdominal pain can be very difficult to assess. The location, quality, duration and description of the pain are exceptionally important for a correct diagnosis. If you have had this pain previously, inform your physician of the diagnosis.

Les douleurs abdominales

Les douleurs abdominales sont difficiles à diagnostiquer. Il est de toute première importance, pour établir un diagnostic correct, de préciser la localisation, le type de douleur, la durée et les caractéristiques de cette douleur. Si vous avez déjà eu des douleurs de ce genre, parlez-en à votre médecin.

Check only those questions to which you answer YES.
Cochez seulement les questions auxquelles vous répondez OUI.

Complaint
Symptômes
❏ I have abdominal pain located here. (Refer to Abdominal Diagram)
    J'ai une douleur abdominale à cet endroit-ci. (Voir le diagramme
    de l'abdomen)
❏ The pain started _____ minutes/hours/days ago.
    La douleur a débuté il y _____ minutes/heures/jours.

Associated symptoms and history
Symptômes associés et informations complémentaires
❏ The pain feels:
    La douleur est:
      ❏ sharp, like a knife.
        aiguë, comme un coup de couteau.
      ❏ dull and aching.
          sourde.
      ❏ crampy.
        comme une crampe.
❏ The pain:
    La douleur:
      ❏ stays in one place. (Demonstrate)
        reste au même endroit. (Démontrer)
      ❏ radiates to my back. (Demonstrate).
        se propage dans le dos. (Démontrer)
      ❏ radiates to my right/left shoulder blades. (Demonstrate)
        se propage dans l'homoplate gauche/droite. (Démontrer)
      ❏ moves throughout my abdomen.
        se déplace dans tout l'abdomen.
      ❏ radiates into my right/left testicle(s).
        se propage dans les droit/gauche testicules.
      ❏ radiates into my groin.
        se propage à l'entre-jambes.
❏ The pain feels better when I:

La douleur s'atténue quand je:
❑ eat food.
    mange.
❑ do not eat food.
    ne mange pas.
❑ vomit.
    vomis.
❑ move my bowels.
    vais à la selle.
❑ curl into a fetal position.
    me mets en position fœtale.
❑ urinate.
    j'urine.
❑ The pain feels worse when I:
Le douleur s'accentue quand je:
❑ eat food.
    ❑ mange.
    do not eat food.
    ne mange pas.
❑ twist my torso back and forth.
    bouge le torse d'avant en arrière.
❑ sit up.
    me redresse d'une position couchée.
❑ take a deep breath.
    j'inspire profondément.
❑ have sexual intercourse.
    j'ai des rapports sexuels.
❑ The pain does not change despite anything I do.
La douleur est constante quoi que je fasse.
❑ The pain started around my umbilicus and then moved toward my
    right lower abdomen. (Refer to Abdominal Diagram)
La douleur a débuté près du nombril et s'est propagée vers le bas
de mon abdomen à droite. (Voir le diagramme de l'abdomen)
❑ I also have:
J'ai aussi:
    ❑ nausea.

des nausées.

❏ vomiting.

des vomissements.

❏ fever. (Refer to Temperature Scale)

de la fièvre. (Voir l'échelle de température)

❏ nausea and vomiting.

des nausées et des vomissements.

❏ diarrhea. (Refer to Diarrhea Section)

la diarrhea. (Voir section diarrhée)

❏ chills.

des frissons.

❏ sweats.

des suées.

❏ shaking so badly I cannot stop.

des convulsions si fortes que je ne peux plus m'arrêter.

❏ I have had my gallbladder removed.

Je me suis fait opérer de la vésicule biliaire.

❏ I have not had my gallbladder removed.

Je ne me suis pas fait opérer de la vésicule biliaire.

❏ I have had surgery on my abdomen. (Refer to Medical History Section)

Je me suis déjà fait opérer de l'abdomen. (Voir antécédents médicaux.)

❏ I have had this pain before. (Refer to Medical History Section)

J'ai déjà eu mal comme cela. (Voir antécédents médicaux)

❏ I have taken these medications. (Show medications)

J'ai pris ces médicaments-ci. (Montrer les médicaments.)

Constipation

Many patients have constipation. This is usually due to dehydration and/or to an underlying medical illnesses (including medications). This section will assist you in providing pertinent information to your physician regarding this complaint.

La constipation

De nombreux patients souffrent de constipation. Celle-ci est généralement due à un phénomène de déshydratation et/ou à des maladies sous-jacentes (et à leurs médicaments). Cette section vous aidera à fournir des informations importantes à votre médecin concernant ce dont vous souffrez.

Check only those questions to which you answer YES.
Cochez seulement les questions auxquelles vous répondez OUI.

Complaint
Symptômes

❏ I am constipated.
   Je suis constipé(e).
❏ I have been constipated for _____ days/weeks.
   Je suis constipé(e) depuis _____ jours/semaines.

Associated symptoms and history
Symptômes associés et informations complémentaires

❏ I have a history of constipation.
   Je souffre de constipation chronique.
❏ I take laxatives regularly for constipation. (Refer to section on Medications)
   Je prends régulièrement des laxatifs pour la constipation. (Voir section medicaments)
❏ The last time I had a normal bowel movement was _____ days/weeks ago.
   La dernière que je suis allé(e) à la selle normalement, c'était il y a_____ jours/semaines.
❏ I have to strain when I move my bowels.
   Il faut que je pousse fort quand je vais à la selle.
❏ I can only eliminate a small amount of feces.
   Je n'arrive à éliminer qu'une petite quantité de matières fécales.
❏ I have noticed that my stools are hard, small and like pellets.
   J'ai constaté que mes selles étaient dures, petites, et comme de petites billes.
❏ I have noticed that my stools are thinner than before.
   J'ai constaté que mes selles sont plus fines qu'avant.
❏ I have noticed streaks of red blood on the outside of the stool.

(Refer to Gastrointestinal Bleeding Section)

J'ai constaté que mes selles contiennent des raies de sang rouge en surface. (Voir la section du saignement gastrointestinal)

❏ I have red blood on the tissue paper. (Refer to Gastrointestinal Bleeding Section)

Il y a du sang rouge sur le papier hygiénique. (Voir la section du saignement gastrointestinal)

❏ I have noticed that blood is mixed into the formed part of the stool.(Refer to Gastrointestinal Bleeding Section)

J'ai constaté que du sang était mélangé au bloc formé par la matière fécale. (Voir la section du saignement gastrointestinal.)

❏ I have black colored stool. (Refer to Gastrointestinal Bleeding Section)

Mes selles sont noires. (Voir la section du saignement gastrointestinal.)

❏ I started a new medication recently. The new medication is

_____.

J'ai récemment commencé un nouveau médicament. Le nouveau médicament s'appelle _____.

❏ I have abdominal pain. (Refer to Abdominal Pain Section)

J'ai une douleur abdominale. (Voir la section des doulours abdominales)

❏ I have nausea.

J'ai la nausée.

❏ I have been vomiting.

J'ai des vomissements.

❏ I have a fever.

J'ai de la fièvre.

❏ I have not been drinking much water lately.

Je n'ai pas bu beaucoup d'eau ces derniers temps.

❏ I have tried these laxatives. (Show laxatives or refer to Medications Section)

J'ai essayé ces laxatifs-ci.

❏ I used enemas.

J'ai fait des lavements.

Diarrhea

Diarrhea is a common problem. Informing the physician of the duration, color, volume (large or small) and other complaints is important for a correct diagnosis. Review the foods that you have eaten recently. Did any taste bad? Have you taken any antibiotics recently (up to three months ago)? Review these questions carefully. Usually stool cultures, abdominal x-rays, and blood work are used to assist in the diagnosis.

La diarrhea

La diarrhée est un problème courant. Il est important d'en préciser à votre médecin la durée, la couleur, le volume (petit ou gros) et tout autre renseignement afin qu'il puisse établir un diagnostic correct. Passez en revue ce que vous avez consommé récemment. Est-ce que quelque chose avait mauvais goût? Avez-vous pris des antibiotiques récemment (au cours des trois derniers mois)? Lisez les questions suivantes attentivement. Généralement, on utilise des cultures de matières fécales, des radiographies abdominales et des analyses de sang pour préciser le diagnostic.

Check only those questions to which you answer YES.
Cochez seulement les questions auxquelles vous répondez OUI.

Complaint
Symptômes
❏ I have diarrhea.
    J'ai la diarrhée.
❏ The diarrhea started _____ minutes/hours/days ago.
    Cette diarrhée a débuté il y a _____ minutes/heures/jours.
❏ I have fever. (Refer to Temperature Scale)
    J'ai de la fièvre. (Voir l'échelle de température)

Associated symptoms and history
Symptômes associés et informations complémentaires
❏ I have diarrhea _____ times per day.
    J'ai la diarrhée _____ fois par jour.
❏ The diarrhea looks:
    La diarrhée:

❏ like it contains red blood. (Refer to Gastrointestinal Bleeding
  Section)
  semble contenir du sang rouge. (Voir la section du saigne
    ment gastrointestinal)
❏ like it contains black material. (Refer to Gastrointestinal
  Bleeding Section)
  semble contenir une substance noire. (Voir la section du
    saignement gastrointestinal)
❏ like water.
  ressemble à de l'eau.
❏ like pus.
  ressemble à du pus.
❏ like poorly formed stools.
  ressemble à des selles mal formées.
❏ like brown water.
  ressemble à de l'eau marron.
❏ yellow.
  est jaune.
❏ green.
  est verte.
❏ I have abdominal pain. (Refer to Abdominal Pain Section)
  J'ai une douleur abdominale. (Voir section douleurs abdominales)
❏ I normally have _____ bowel movements per day.
  Je vais normalement à la selle _____ fois par jour.
❏ I have nausea. (Refer to Nausea Section)
  J'ai la nausée. (Voir section nausée)
❏ I have been vomiting. (Refer to Vomiting Section)
  J'ai des vomissements. (Voir section vomissements)
❏ I have had aches and pains in my muscles and joints.
  J'ai des courbatures et des douleurs dans les muscles et les
    articulations.
❏ Others in my party have also been ill with similar problems.
  D'autres personnes dans mon groupe ont aussi été malades avec
    des problèmes similaires.
❏ I know of no others who are ill.
  Je ne connais personne d'autre qui ait été malade.

❑ I ate no food which tasted bad.
  Je n'ai pas mangé d'aliments qui avaient mauvais goût.
❑ Before my diarrhea started, I ate:
  Avant d'avoir la diarrhée, j'avais mangé:
    ❑ poultry that tasted bad.
      de la volaille qui avait mauvais goût.
    ❑ uncooked beef which tasted bad.
      du bœuf cru qui avait mauvais goût.
    ❑ uncooked fish which tasted bad.
      du poisson cru qui avait mauvais goût.
    ❑ cooked beef which tasted bad.
      du bœuf cuit qui avait mauvais goût.
    ❑ cooked fish which tasted bad.
      du poisson cuit qui avait mauvais goût.
    ❑ milk products which tasted bad.
      des produits laitiers qui avaient mauvais goût.
    ❑ cheese which tasted bad.
      du fromage qui avait mauvais goût.
❑ I have traveled to: _____.
  (List cities and/or countries)
  Je suis allé(e) à/en (aux) _____.
  (Faire la liste des villes et/ou pays)
❑ I have not taken any antibiotics for the past three months.
  Je n'ai pris aucun antibiotique au cours des trois derniers mois.
❑ I took antibiotics about _____ weeks ago.
  J'ai pris des antibiotiques il y a environ _____ semaines.
❑ I have a milk allergy.
  Je suis allergique au lait.
❑ I have tried limiting my diet.
  J'ai essayé de manger moins.
❑ I have tried anti-diarrhea agents. I have used _____.
  J'ai essayé des anti-diarrhéiques. J'ai pris _____.
❑ I have been avoiding milk products.
  J'ai évité les produits laitiers.
❑ I have not tried any specific treatments.
  Je n'ai pas essayé de traitement particulier.

Gastrointestinal Bleeding

Gastrointestinal (GI) bleeding can be severe. The general appearance of the blood is extremely important. The first assessment of the location of the GI bleeding is divided into upper or lower GI tracts. The upper GI tract is generally the stomach and the first part of the small intestine. Feces may be either red or black (tarry appearing, foul smelling, thick stools). The presence of red blood also may indicate lower GI bleeding. If you are lightheaded or have had an episode of passing out and you have red blood in your feces, rapid upper GI bleeding may be present. Lower GI bleeding is usually painless, associated with red blood, and usually does not have a black foul-smelling stool.

A history of previous problems of GI bleeding is very important as is any history of liver disease or bleeding problems.

Les saignements gastro-intestinaux

Les saignements gastro-intestinaux peuvent être graves. L'aspect général du sang est important. La première évaluation de la localisation de ces saignements gastro-intestinaux est divisée entre les systèmes gastro-intestinaux supérieur et inférieur. Le système gastro-intestinal supérieur comprend généralement l'estomac et la première partie de l'estomac. Le sang dans les matières fécales peut être rouge ou noir (selles épaisses, nauséabondes, ayant l'aspect du goudron). La présence de sang rouge peut aussi indiquer un saignement gastro-intestinal inférieur. Si vous avez la tête qui tourne ou si vous vous êtes évanoui(e) et que vous avez du sang rouge, vous pouvez avoir un saignement gastro-intestinal supérieur rapide. Un saignement gastro-intestinal inférieur est généralement indolore; il est lié à du sang rouge et les selles ne sont généralement ni noires ni nauséabondes.

Il est très important de préciser si vous souffrez de saignements gastro-intestinaux chroniques ou de toute autre maladie chronique concernant le foie ou se caractérisant par des saignements anormaux.

Check only those questions to which you answer YES.
Cochez seulement les questions auxquelles vous répondez OUI.

Complaint
Symptômes

❏ I have been vomiting blood.
   Je vomis du sang.
❏ The problem started _____ minutes/hours/days ago.
   Ce problème a débuté il y a _____ minutes/heures/jours.
❏ The vomit looks like:
   Le vomi ressemble à:
   ❏ red blood.
      du sang rouge.
   ❏ little black flecks that look like coffee grounds.
      des petites particules noires qui ressemblent à du café moulu.
❏ I have a fever. (Refer to Temperature Scale)
   J'ai de la fièvre. (Voir l'échelle de température)

Associated symptoms and history
Symptômes associés et informations complémentaires

❏ I have been lightheaded.
   J'ai la tête qui tourne.
❏ I nearly passed out.
   J'ai failli m'évanouir.
❏ I have passed out.
   Je me suis évanoui(e).
❏ I get lightheaded when I stand up or rise from bed.
   J'ai la tête qui tourne quand je me redresse ou me lève de mon
      lit.
❏ I have abdominal pain. (Refer to Abdominal Pain Section)
   J'ai une douleur abdominale. (Voir section douleurs abdominales)
❏ I have been passing black bowel movements.
   Mes selles sont noires.
❏ I have had ulcers in the past.
   J'ai déjà eu des ulcères.

❏ I have never had ulcers.

Je n'ai jamais eu d'ulcères.

❏ I take aspirin.

Je prends de l'aspirine.

❏ I take medications for joint pain. (Show medications)

Je prends des médicaments contre les douleurs articulaires.

(Montrer ces medicaments)

❏ I drink alcoholic beverages. I usually drink:

Je bois de l'alsool. Je bois généralement:

  ❏ beer.

    de la bière

  ❏ wine.

    du vin.

  ❏ liquor.

    des alcools forts.

❏ I usually drink about _____ drinks per day.

Je bois généralement environ _____ fois par jour.

❏ My last drink was _____ hours/days ago.

La dernière fois que j'ai bu, c'était il y a _____ heures/jours.

❏ I have had kidney problems in the past. (Refer to Medical History Section).

J'ai déjà eu des problèmes de reins. (Voir antécédents médicaux)

❏ I have had problems with my liver.

J'ai déjà eu des problèmes de foie.

❏ I bleed easily.

Je saigne facilement.

❏ I have a family history of easy bleeding.

On saigne facilement dans ma famille.

❏ I take the following medications:

Je prends les médicaments suivants:

(No translations are given because the French spelling of the medications are the same as or very similar to the English spelling.)

  ❏ Ranitidine (Zantac)

  ❏ Famotidine (Pepcid)

- ❏ Cimetidine (Tagamet)
- ❏ Nizatidine (Axid)
- ❏ Omeprazole (Prilosec)
- ❏ Pentaprazole (Protonix)
- ❏ Esomeprazole (Nexium)
- ❏ Rabeprazole (Aciphex)
- ❏ Pantoprazole (Protonix)

❏ I have liver disease.
J'ai une maladie du foie.

❏ I have had bleeding from the esophagus in the past.
J'ai déjà eu des saignements œsophagiens.

❏ I have bleeding from the esophagus due to reflux disease.
J'ai un saignement œsophagien dû à un reflux gastro-œsophagien.

❏ I have bleeding from the esophagus due to ruptured blood vessels.
J'ai un saignement œsophagien dû à la rupture de vaisseaux sanguins.

❏ The last time I had bleeding was _____.
La dernière que j'ai saigné, c'était _____.

❏ I have taken these medications. (Show medications)
J'ai pris ces médicaments. (Montrer ces medicaments)

Jaundice

Jaundice is a condition where the white part of the eyes becomes yellow. As the condition progresses, the skin becomes yellow as well. Urine may turn yellow. The feces may also turn to a white color. The condition may or may not be associated with gallstones. In either case, the liver is functioning abnormally.

La jaunisse

La jaunisse est une maladie qui rend jaune la partie blanche des yeux. Au fur et à mesure que la maladie progresse, la peau devient jaune également. L'urine peut devenir jaune. Les matières fécales peuvent aussi prendre une couleur blanche. La maladie peut être ou non associée à des calculs biliaires. Dans les deux cas, le foie fonctionne de façon anormale.

Check only those questions to which you answer YES.
Cochez seulement les questions auxquelles vous répondez OUI.

Complaint
Symptômes
❑ I am yellow.
   J'ai le teint jaune.
❑ This started _____ hours/days/weeks ago.
   Cela a débuté il y a _____ heures/jours/semaines.
❑ I have a fever. (Refer to Temperature Scale)
   J'ai de la fièvre. (Voir l'échelle de température)

Associated symptoms and history
Symptômes associés et informations complémentaires
❑ I itch.
   Cela me démange.
❑ I have pain in my abdomen. (Refer to Abdominal Pain Section)
   J'ai mal à l'abdomen. (Voir section douleurs abdominales)
❑ I have noticed that my urine has become tea colored. This occurred
   _____ days/weeks ago.
   J'ai constaté que mes urines étaient devenues de la couleur du
   thé. Cela s'est produit il y a _____ jours/semaines.
❑ I have noticed that my stools are a white or light tan color. This
   occurred _____ days ago.
   J'ai constaté que mes selles sont blanches ou marron clair. Cela
   s'est produit il y a _____ jours/semaines.
❑ I have been using recreational drugs.
   Je consomme des drogues douces.
❑ I have been drinking alcohol.
   Je bois de l'alcool.
❑ My last drink was _____ hours/days/weeks ago.
   La dernière fois que j'ai bu de l'alcool, c'était il y a _____
   heures/jours/mois.
❑ I have been close to an individual who has hepatitis.
   J'ai été en contact avec un individu qui a une hépatite.
❑ I have had sexual intercourse with someone who has hepatitis.

J'ai eu des rapports sexuels avec quelqu'un qui a une hépatite.
❏ I have had my hepatitis A vaccine.
  Je me suis fait vacciner contre l'hépatite A.
❏ I have had my Hepatitis B vaccine.
  Je me suis fait vacciner contre l'hépatite B.
❏ I have Hepatitis C.
  J'ai l'hépatite C.
❏ I have been told I have had abnormal liver function tests.
  On m'a dit que mes tests montraient un fonctionnement anormal
  du foie.
❏ I have taken a new medication recently. (Show medication)
  J'ai récemment pris un nouveau médicament. (Montrer
  médicament)
❏ I have eaten some food that did not taste fresh. This meal was
  _____hours/days/weeks ago.
  J'ai mangé quelque chose qui avait mauvais goût. C'était il y a
  _____ heures/jours/semaines.
❏ I ate seafood recently.
  J'ai mangé des fruits de mer récemment.
❏ I have been sexually active recently.
  J'ai eu des rapports sexuels récemment.

Swallowing Difficulties

Problems swallowing are not uncommon. Usually, a history of heart-burn or GERD precedes the acute problem. Informing the physician of the onset of the problem and the type of food that you ate is important.
    An endoscopic procedure may be required for resolution of this problem.

Les problèmes de deglutition

Les problèmes de déglutition sont fréquents. Généralement, des brûlures d'estomac récurrentes et un reflux gastro-œsophagien chronique précèdent la crise aiguë. Il est important de préciser au médecin à quel moment le problème a débuté et quel type de nourri-ture vous avez consommé.
    Une procédure endoscopique peut s'avérer nécessaire pour résoudre ce problème.

Check only those questions to which you answer YES.
Cochez seulement les questions auxquelles vous répondez OUI.

Complaint
Symptômes
❏ I have food stuck in my throat.
   J'ai de la nourriture coincée dans la gorge.
❏ I ate a piece of meat.
   J'ai mangé un morceau de viande.
❏ I ate chicken.
   J'ai mangé du poulet.
❏ I ate fish.
   J'ai mangé du poisson.
❏ This happened _____ minutes/hours ago.
   Cela s'est passé il y a _____ minutes/heures.
❏ I am able to swallow my saliva.
   J'arrive à avaler ma salive.
❏ I am unable to swallow my saliva.
   Je n'arrive pas à avaler ma salive.
❏ I have had food lodge in my throat in the past.
   J'ai déjà eu de la nourriture coincée dans la gorge.
❏ I have had problems with heartburn in the past.
   J'ai déjà eu des brûlures d'estomac.
❏ I have had my esophagus dilated in the past.
   J'ai déjà eu l'œsophage dilaté.
❏ The last time I had my esophagus dilated was _____.
   La dernière fois que j'ai eu l'œsophage dilaté, c'était _____.
❏ I have difficulty swallowing food.
   J'ai du mal à avaler de la nourriture.
❏ This happens primarily with solid food.
   C'est le cas essentiellement avec les aliments solides.
❏ This happens primarily with liquids.
   C'est le cas essentiellement avec les liquides.
❏ This happens with both solids and liquids.
   C'est le cas avec les aliments solides et les liquides.
❏ This happens when I drink hot/cold/both liquids.

C'est le cas quand je bois des liquides chauds/froids/les deux.

❏ I have a history of heartburn.

J'ai des brûlures d'estomac récurrentes.

❏ I have painful swallowing. The food passes through my esophagus but it causes pain while passing.

J'ai du mal à avaler.La nourriture passe bien par l'œsophage mais cela me fait mal quand elle passe.

❏ I have tried the following medications _____.

J'ai essayé les médicaments suivants _____.

❏ I have tried to vomit.

J'ai essayé de vomir.

GENITOURINARY TRACT (URINARY TRACT, KIDNEYS AND GENITALIA)

VOIES GÉNITO-URINAIRES (VOIES URINAIRES, RÉNAUX ET ORGANES GÉNITAUX)

Blood in the Urine (Hematuria)

Bloody urine is usually associated with infection, stones, or tumors of the GU tract. The following will be useful in providing pertinent information to your physician regarding this complaint.

Please be sure that the forms regarding your medical history, current medications, allergies, etc. have been filled out completely. The information in this section is invaluable to all health care providers.

Le sang dans les urines (hématurie)

Le sang dans les urines est généralement lié à des infections, des calculs et des tumeurs dans les voies génito-urinaires. Les questions suivantes seront utiles pour fournir des renseignements importants à votre médecin concernant ce don't vous souffrez.

Check only those questions to which you answer YES.
Cochez seulement les questions auxquelles vous répondez OUI.

Complaint
Symptômes

❑ My urine is red.
  Mes urines sont rouges.
❑ This problem has been present for _____ hours/days.
  J'ai ce problème depuis _____ heures/jours.

Associated symptoms and history
Symptômes associés et informations complémentaires

❑ The last time I saw normal colored urine was _____ hours/days
  ago.
  Le dernière fois que j'ai constaté que mes urines étaient de
  couleur normale, c'était il y a _____ heures/jours.
❑ I have pain when I urinate.
  Cela me fait mal quand j'urine.

❏ I have had kidney stones in the past.
  J'ai déjà eu des calculs rénaux.
❏ I have had a bladder tumor in the past.
  J'ai déjà eu une tumeur à la vessie.
❏ I have trouble initiating urination.
  J'ai du mal à commencer d'uriner.
❏ I have pain in my right/left/both testicles.
  J'ai mal au testicule droit/gauche/aux deux.
❏ I have a fever.
  J'ai de la fièvre.
❏ I have been nauseated.
  J'ai la nausée.
❏ I have been vomiting.
  J'ai des vomissements.
❏ I have a discharge from my penis/vagina.
  J'ai un écoulement du pénis/des pertes vaginales.
❏ I have lost weight recently. I have lost _____ pounds. (2.2 pounds =
  1 kilogram)
  J'ai perdu du poids récemment. J'ai perdu _____ kilos.

Kidney Stones

This section is designed to report the information regarding kidney stones. Kidney stones may present with blood in the urine. This may be either red blood that is easily visible (gross hematuria) or microscopic amounts of blood. If you have urine that is bright or dark red or tea colored, kidney stones may be present. The pain associated with kidney stones may start in the right or left upper abdomen and then progress (or radiate) into the flanks (left or right), the testicles or both. If you have had kidney stones before, fill out this section. If you are unsure about the nature of your abdominal pain, fill out the section on Abdominal Pain. Review this section and complete it if necessary. Always complete as many sections as you believe are applicable. Information is always useful to the physician.

Les calculs rénaux

Cette section a été conçue pour fournir des renseignements concernant les calculs rénaux.

Check only those questions to which you answer YES.
Cochez seulement les questions auxquelles vous répondez OUI.

Complaint
Symptômes

❏ I am passing a kidney stone.
   J'évacue par les urines un calcul rénal.
❏ I have had kidney stones in the past.
   J'ai déjà eu des calculs rénaux.
❏ I had my first kidney stones at _____ years of age.
   J'ai eu mon premier calcul rénal à l'âge de _____ ans.
❏ I have passed one/few/many kidney stones.
   J'ai déjà évacué par les urines un/quelques/beaucoup de calcul(s)
   renal(aux).
❏ The stones were _____ mm in size. (Describe size of stone or refer
   to Metric Conversion Chart)
   Les calculs mesuraient _____ mms. (Décrire la taille du calcul)
❏ When I have an attack, I usually pass several stones.
   Quand je fais une crise, j'évacue par les urines plusieurs calculs.
❏ I have had:
   J'ai déjà eu:
   ❏ calcium oxalate stones.
      des calculs d'oxalate de calcium.
   ❏ struvite stones.
      des calculs struviques.
   ❏ cystine stones.
      des calculs cystiniques.
   ❏ staghorn calculi.
      des calculs coralliformes.
   ❏ I don't know what type of stones I have had in the past.
      Je ne sais pas quel type de calculs j'ai déjà eu.
❏ I have had:
   J'ai déjà eu:
   ❏ extra-corporeal shock wave lithotripsy (ESWL).
      une lithotrypsie extra-corporelle par ondes de choc.
   ❏ surgery.

une opération.

❑ removal via my penis/urethra.

une opération par les voies naturelles (pénis/urêtre).

❑ a stent (plastic tube) placed in my ureter.

une sonde (un tube en plastique) placé dans l'urêtre.

❑ I have never had any surgery or intervention to remove the stones.

Je n'ai jamais eu d'opération ou d'intervention chirurgicale pour retirer des calculs.

❑ I have the following problems:

J'ai les problèmes suivants:

   ❑ high calcium levels in my blood.

   une calcémie élevée.

   ❑ a history of a tumor. (Refer to Medical History Section)

   des tumeurs récurrentes. (Voir antécédents médicaux)

   ❑ hyperparathyroidism.

   de l'hyperparathyroïdie.

   ❑ hyperthyroidism (increased thyroid activity).

   de l'hyperthyroïdie (activité accrue de la glande thyroïde).

   ❑ gout.

   de la goutte.

   ❑ Crohn's Disease.

   la maladie de Crohn.

   ❑ kidney disease.

   une maladie des reins.

❑ I have not been drinking enough fluids lately.

Je n'ai pas bu assez de fluides ces derniers temps.

❑ I have been exercising lately.

J'ai fait de l'exercice ces derniers temps.

❑ I eat a lot of meat.

Je mange beaucoup de viande.

❑ I have been eating a lot of salt lately.

J'ai mangé très salé ces derniers temps.

Sexually Transmitted Diseases: Male

This section is designed to report the information regarding sexually transmitted diseases.

Understandably, this area is quite difficult to pursue. It is imperative that you be as accurate as possible. Since sexual activity is common, recent events are very important. Pay attention to this history first but be as complete as you can with your answers.

Les maladies sexuellement transmissibles: chez l'homme
Cette section a été conçue pour fournir des renseignements concernant les maladies sexuellement transmissibles.

Il est bien entendu que ce domaine est très délicat à explorer. Il est impératif que vous répondiez aussi précisément que possible. Etant donné que l'activité sexuelle est une pratique courante, les événements récents qui se sont produits sont très importants. Veuillez les considérer avec une attention toute particulière et soyez aussi précis que possible dans vos réponses.

Check only those questions to which you answer YES.
Cochez seulement les questions auxquelles vous répondez OUI.

Complaint
Symptômes
❏ I have a discharge from my penis.
 J'ai un écoulement du pénis.
❏ I have rectal itching.
 J'ai des démangeaisons rectales.
❏ I have a wart in my genital area.
 J'ai une verrue aux parties génitales.
❏ I have an ulcer in my genital area.
 J'ai un ulcère aux parties génitales.
❏ This problem has been present for _____ hours/days/weeks.
 J'ai ce problème depuis _____ heures/jours/semaines.
❏ I have a sex partner who has a sexually transmitted disease. I have been told I need to be evaluated for the same problem.
 J'ai un partenaire sexuel qui a une maladie sexuellement transmissible. On m'a dit que je devais consulter un médecin pour le même problème.

Associated symptoms and history
Symptômes associés et informations complémentaires

❏ I am heterosexual/bisexual/homosexual.
 Je suis hétérosexuel/bisexuel/homosexuel.

❏ I have a fever. (Refer to Temperature Scale)
 J'ai de la fièvre. (Voir l'échelle de température)

❏ I have a burning sensation when I urinate.
 Cela me brûle quand j'urine.

❏ I have recently had sexual relations with a man/woman/both.
 J'ai eu récemment des rapports sexuels avec un homme/une
  femme/les deux.

❏ During the past 4 weeks, I have had sexual relations with
  _____ different partners.
 Durant les 4 dernières semaines, j'ai eu des rapports sexuels avec
  _____ partenaires différents.

❏ I have used condoms.
 J'ai utilisé des préservatifs.

❏ I did not use a condom.
 Je n'ai pas utilisé de préservatifs.

❏ I have given oral sex.
 J'ai pratiqué une fellation/un cunnilingus.

❏ I have received oral sex.
 On m'a fait une fellation.

❏ I have given anal sex.
 J'ai sodomisé mon partenaire.

❏ I have received anal sex.
 J'ai été sodomisé.

❏ I have had vaginal intercourse.
 J'ai eu des rapports sexuels avec pénétration vaginale.

❏ I have had sexual relations with prostitutes.
 J'ai eu des rapports sexuels avec des prostitué(e)s.

❏ I have HIV.
 Je suis séropositif.

❏ I have AIDS.
 J'ai le sida.

❑ My partner did/did not use a condom.

Mon partenaire a utilisé un préservatif/n'a pas utilisé de préservatifs.

❑ I have had sexually transmitted diseases in the past.

J'ai déjà eu des maladies sexuellement transmissibles.

❑ I use recreational drugs.

Je consomme des drogues douces.

❑ I drink alcohol.

Je bois de l'alcool.

❑ I have had a rash. (Show)

J'ai de l'urticaire. (Montrer)

❑ I have joint pain.

J'ai une douleur articulaire.

❑ I have diarrhea. (Refer to Diarrhea Section)

J'ai la diarrhée. (Voir la section diarrhea)

❑ I have new bumps here. (Refer to Groin Diagrams)

J'ai de nouvelles déformations à l'aine. (Voir les diagrammes de l'aine)

❑ These are/are not tender.

Elles sont sensibles/ne sont pas sensibles.

❑ I have traveled to third-world countries recently.

J'ai voyagé dans des pays du Tiers-Monde récemment.

❑ I have herpes.

J'ai de l'herpès.

❑ I have pain in my right/left/both testicle(s).

J'ai mal au testicule droit/gauche/aux deux.

❑ I have not seen blood in my urine.

Je n'ai pas constaté la présence de sang dans mes urines.

Sexually Transmitted Diseases: Female

This section is designed to report the information regarding sexually transmitted diseases.

Understandably, this area is quite difficult to pursue. It is imperative that you be as accurate as possible. Since sexual activity is common, recent events are very important. Pay attention to this history first but be as complete as you can with your answers.

Les maladies sexuellement transmissibles: chez la femme
Cette section a été conçue pour fournir des renseignements concernant les maladies sexuellement transmissibles.
Il est bien entendu que ce domaine est très délicat à explorer. Il est impératif que vous répondiez aussi précisément que possible. Etant donné que l'activité sexuelle est une pratique courante, les événements récents qui se sont produits sont très importants. Veuillez les considérer avec une attention toute particulière et soyez aussi préciss que possible dans vos réponses.

Check only those questions to which you answer YES.
Cochez seulement les questions auxquelles vous répondez OUI.

Complaint
Symptômes
❑ I have a discharge from my vagina.
  J'ai des pertes vaginales.
❑ The discharge from my vagina is:
  Mes pertes vaginales sont:
  ❑ white.
    blanches.
  ❑ yellow.
    jaunes.
  ❑ brown.
    marron.
❑ I have vaginal itching.
  J'ai des démangeaisons vaginales.
❑ I have rectal itching.
  J'ai des démangeaisons rectales.
❑ I have a wart in my genital area. (Show)
  J'ai une verrue dans les parties génitales. (Montrer)
❑ I have an ulcer in my genital area.
  J'ai un ulcère dans les parties génitales.
❑ This problem has been present for _____ hours/days/weeks.
  J'ai ce problème depuis _____ heures/jours/semaines.
❑ I have a partner who has a sexually transmitted disease. I have been

told I need to be evaluated for the same problem. I last had
sexual intercourse with this individual on _____. (date)
J'ai un partenaire qui a une maladie sexuellement transmissible.
On m'a dit qu'il fallait que je consulte un médecin pour le
même problème. Mon dernier rapport sexuel avec cet individu
date de _____.

Associated symptoms and history
Symptômes associés et informations complémentaires
❑ I am heterosexual/bisexual/lesbian.
  Je suis hétérosexuelle/bisexuelle/lesbienne.
❑ I have a fever.
  J'ai de la fièvre.
❑ I have a burning sensation when I urinate.
  Cela me brûle quand j'urine.
❑ I have been having sexual relations with a man/woman/both.
  J'ai eu des rapports sexuels avec un homme/une femme/les deux.
❑ During the past four weeks, I have had sexual relations with _____
  different partners.
  Durant les 4 dernières semaines, j'ai eu des rapports sexuels avec
  _____ partenaires différents.
❑ My partners have used condoms.
  Mes partenaires ont utilisé des préservatifs.
❑ I have given oral sex.
  J'ai pratiqué une fellation/un cunnilingus.
❑ I have received oral sex.
  On m'a fait un cunnilingus.
❑ I have received anal sex.
  Je me suis fait sodomiser.
❑ I have had vaginal intercourse.
  J'ai eu un rapport sexuel avec pénétration.
❑ I have HIV.
  Je suis séropositive.
❑ I have AIDS.
  J'ai le sida.
❑ My partner did/did not use a condom.

Mon partenaire a utilisé un préservatif/ n'a pas utilisé de
préservatif.
❑ My last menstrual period was _____. (date)
Mes dernières règles remontent à _____. (date)
❑ My last menstrual period was:
Mes dernières règles étaient:
  ❑ normal.
    normales.
  ❑ light.
    peu abondantes.
  ❑ heavy.
    abondantes.
❑ I have had sexually transmitted diseases in the past.
  J'ai déjà eu des maladies sexuellement transmissibles.
❑ I use recreational drugs.
  Je consomme des drogues douces.
❑ I drink alcohol.
  Je bois de l'alcool.
❑ I have had a rash.
  J'ai de l'urticaire.
❑ I have joint pain.
  J'ai des douleurs articulaires.
❑ I have diarrhea. (Refer to Diarrhea Section)
  J'ai la diarrhea. (Voir la section diarrhea)
❑ I have new bumps here. (Refer to Groin Diagrams)
  J'ai de nouvelles déformations à l'aine. (Voir les diagrammes de
    l'aine)
❑ These are/are not tender.
  Elles sont sensibles/ne sont pas sensibles.
❑ I have traveled to third-world countries recently.
  J'ai récemment voyagé dans des pays du Tiers-Monde.
❑ I have herpes.
  J'ai de l'herpès.
❑ I have douched recently.
  Je me suis récemment fait une douche intra-vaginale.

❏ I have not seen blood in my urine.

Je n'ai pas constaté la présence de sang dans mes urines.

Testicular Pain

Testicular pain may be related to urinary tract stones, infection, or tumors. If you have a history of urinary tract stones, a further review of that section would be useful.

The following will be useful in providing pertinent information to your physician regarding this complaint.

Les douleurs testiculaires

Les douleurs testiculaires peuvent être liées à des calculs, des infections ou des tumeurs dans les voies urinaires. Si vous avez des antécédents en matière de calculs dans les voies urinaires, il vous serait utile de consulter cette section de manière approfondie.

Les questions ci-dessous seront utiles pour fournir à votre médecin des informations importantes sur ce dont vous souffrez.

Check only those questions to which you answer YES.
Cochez seulement les questions auxquelles vous répondez OUI.

Complaint
Symptômes

❏ I have pain in my right/left/both testicle(s).

J'ai mal au testicule droit/gauche/aux deux testicules.

❏ The pain started _____ minutes/hours/days ago.

J'ai mal depuis _____ minutes/heures/jours.

Associated symptoms and history
Symptômes associés et informations complémentaires

❏ The pain started suddenly.

J'ai eu mal tout à coup.

❏ The pain started gradually.

J'ai eu mal progressivement.

❏ The pain is a dull aching sensation.

La douleur est sourde.

❏ The pain stays in the right/left/both testicle(s).

La douleur reste dans le testicule droit/gauche/dans les deux testicules.

❑ The pain radiates to the right/left/both flanks.
La douleur se propage au flanc droit/gauche/aux deux flancs.

❑ My testicle(s) is/are swollen.
J'ai le(s) testicule(s) enflés.

❑ I have had similar pain in the past.
J'ai déjà eu mal comme cela.

❑ I have had trauma to the right/left/both testicle.
J'ai déjà eu un traumatisme au testicule droit/gauche/aux deux testicules.

❑ I have had pain when I urinate. (Complete the Urinary Tract Section)
J'ai mal quand j'urine. (Compléter la section voies urinaires)

❑ I have a fever.
J'ai de la fièvre.

❑ I have been lifting heavy objects.
J'ai porté des objets lourds.

❑ I have been having sexual relations recently.
J'ai eu des rapports sexuels récemment.

❑ I use a condom.
J'ai utilisé un préservatif.

❑ I have had sexual relations with persons I don't know well.
J'ai eu des rapports sexuels avec des personnes que je ne connais pas très bien.

Urinary Tract Infection

This section is designed to report the information regarding urinary tract problems. Most of the following focuses on urinary tract infections and bleeding from the urinary tract.

Infections des voies urinaires

Cette section a été conçue pour fournir des renseignements sur les problèmes des voies urinaires. La plupart des questions ci-dessous concernent les infections des voies urinaires et les saignements des voies urinaires.

Check only those questions to which you answer YES.
Cochez seulement les questions auxquelles vous répondez OUI.

Complaint
Symptômes

❏ I have been having difficulty urinating.
  J'ai du mal à uriner.
❏ I have a fever. (Refer to Temperature Scale)
  J'ai de la fièvre. (Voir l'échelle de température)
❏ This problem has been present for _____minutes/hours/days/weeks.
  J'ai ce problème depuis _____ minutes/heures/jours/semaines.

Associated symptoms and history
Symptômes associés et informations complémentaires

❏ I urinate in small volumes.
  J'urine en petites quantités.
❏ I urinate frequently.
  J'urine fréquemment.
❏ I urinate at night.
  J'urine la nuit.
❏ I have painful urination.
  J'ai mal quand j'urine.
❏ The pain is present when I start to urinate.
  J'ai mal dès que je commence à uriner.
❏ The pain is present throughout the process of urination.
  J'ai mal pendant tout le temps où j'urine.
❏ The pain is present at the end of urination.
  J'ai mal quand je termine d'uriner.
❏ The last time I urinated was _____ minutes/hours/days ago.
  La dernière fois que j'ai uriné, c'était il y a _____
  minutes/heures/jours.
❏ I have abdominal pain. (Refer to Abdominal Pain Section)
  J'ai une douleur abdominale. (Voir section douleurs abdominales)
❏ I have had problems with my bladder in the past.
  J'ai déjà eu des problèmes de vessie.
❏ This problem has occurred before. (Refer to Medical History
  Section)

J'ai déjà eu ce problème. (Voir antécédents médicaux)

❑ I do not seem to be able to completely empty my bladder.
On dirait que je n'arrive pas à vider complètement ma vessie.

❑ I have seen blood in my urine.
J'ai du sang dans les urines.

❑ I have blood in my urine when I have my menstrual period.
J'ai du sang dans les urines quand j'ai mes règles.

❑ I am having my menstrual period now.
J'ai mes règles en ce moment.

❑ I am passing clots of blood in my urine.
J'évacue des caillots de sang dans mes urines.

❑ When I urinate, I feel like I must urinate immediately.
Quand j'urine, j'ai l'impression qu'il faut que j'urine
immédiatement.

❑ I have a discharge from my penis/vagina. (Refer to Sexually
Transmitted Disease Section)
J'ai un écoulement du pénis/des pertes vaginales. (Voir les
maladies transmises sexuellment)

❑ I have pain in my back. (Refer to Back Diagrams)
J'ai mal au dos. (Voir les diagrammes du dos)

❑ The pain is located on the right/left/both sides.
J'ai mal au côté droit/gauche/des deux côtés.

❑ I have been losing weight.
J'ai perdu du poids.

❑ I have been coughing up blood.
Je crache du sang.

❑ I have been exposed to chemicals lately.
J'ai été récemment en contact avec des produits chimiques.

❑ I have bruised easily lately.
J'attrape des bleus facilement depuis quelque temps.

❑ I have been having joint pain recently.
J'ai des douleurs articulaires depuis quelque temps.

❑ I have been traveling recently in _____.
(city/country)
Je suis récemment allé(e) à/en/aux _____.
(ville/pays)

❑ I have a history of high blood pressure.
  J'ai des problèmes chroniques de tension artérielle élevée.
❑ I have had a rash lately. (Show the rash)
  J'ai de l'urticaire depuis quelque temps. (Montrer cette urticaire)
❑ I began having difficulty urinating after sexual intercourse.
  J'ai commencé à avoir du mal à uriner après un rapport sexuel.
❑ I was recently married.
  Je me suis marié(e) récemment.
❑ I have a thick white discharge from my vagina.
  J'ai des pertes vaginales blanches et épaisses.
❑ I have a thin watery discharge from my vagina.
  J'ai des pertes vaginales liquides et peu épaisses.
❑ I have been urinating frequently.
  J'urine fréquemment.
❑ I have been urinating large volumes of urine.
  J'urine en quantité abondante.
❑ I have been very thirsty lately.
  J'ai très soif depuis quelque temps.
❑ I prefer ice water.
  Je préfère l'eau glacée.
❑ I take lithium.
  Je prends du lithium.
❑ I have had head trauma recently. (Refer to Head Diagram)
  J'ai récemment eu un traumatisme crânien. (Voir les diagrammes
    de la tête)
❑ I have a history of a tumor. (Refer to Medical History)
  J'ai des tumeurs récurrentes. (Voir antécédents médicaux)
❑ I take these medications. (Refer to Medical History)
  Je prends ces médicaments-ci. (Voir antécédents médicaux)
❑ I have had kidney stones in the past. (Refer to Medical History)
  J'ai déjà eu des calculs dans les reins. (Voir antécédents
    médicaux)
❑ I have had:
  J'ai déjà eu:
    ❑ extra-corporeal shock wave lithotripsy (ESWL).
      une lithotrypsie extra-corporelle par ondes de choc.

❏ surgery.
   une opération.
❏ removal via my penis/vagina.
   une opération par les voies naturelles pénis/vagin.
❏ a stent placed in my ureter.
   une sonde placée dans l'urêtre.
❏ I have never had any surgery or intervention to remove the stones.
   Je n'ai jamais subi d'opération ou d'intervention chirurgicale
   pour retirer des calculs.
❏ I have:
   J'ai:
      ❏ calcium oxalate stones.
         des calculs d'oxalate de calcium.
      ❏ struvite stones.
         des calculs struviques.
      ❏ cystine stones.
         des calculs cystiniques
      ❏ staghorn calculi.
         des calculs coralliformes.
❏ I don't know what types of stones I have had in the past.
   Je ne sais pas quel type de calculs j'ai déjà eu.
❏ I have abdominal pain. (Refer to Abdominal Pain Section)
   J'ai une douleur abdominale. (Voir section douleurs abdominales)
❏ The pain is sharp.
   La douleur est aiguê.
❏ The pain is dull.
   La douleur est sourde.
❏ The pain radiates into my groin.
   La douleur se propage à l'entre-jambes.
❏ The pain is always present but seems to get better and worse.
   J'ai mal en permanence mais avec des hauts et des bas.
❏ There is nothing I can do to improve the pain.
   Je ne peux rien faire pour soulager la douleur.
❏ I have a poor urinary stream.
   J'a un débit urinaire déficient.
❏ I have dribbling of the urine at the end of voiding.

J'ai des gouttelettes d'urine qui apparaissent spontanément quand j'ai fini d'uriner.

❑ I have flank pain on the right/left/both sides.

J'ai mal au flanc droit/gauche/aux deux flancs.

❑ The pain starts in the flank and radiates forward into my abdomen. (Refer to Abdominal Diagram)

La douleur commence dans le flanc et se propage dans l'abdomen. (Voir le diagramme de l'abdomen)

❑ I have been drinking less fluid than usual.

Je bois moins de fluides que d'habitude.

❑ I have been exercising a lot.

Je fais beaucoup d'exercice.

Urinary Retention (Inability to Urinate)

Urinary retention may be a slow or acute problem. Pain may not be present when the obstruction to the urinary outflow tract is a slowly progressive process. On the other hand, acute obstruction usually presents with pain that may be severe. Often an ultrasound of the abdomen will be performed. A catheter is usually placed into the urethra in order to relieve the obstruction. Obstructive lesions may be either congenital or acquired.

Rétention d'urine (incapacité à uriner)

La rétention d'urine peut être un problème qui survient lentement ou se développe très rapidement. Lorsque l'obstruction de la voie urinaire survient lentement et progressivement, cela n'est pas nécessairement douloureux. En revanche, une obstruction massive entraîne des douleurs qui peuvent être très importantes. Dans ce cas, on pratiquera souvent un ultrason (échographie) de l'abdomen. Un cathéter est généralement placé dans l'urêtre afin de soulager l'obstruction. Les lésions obstructives peuvent être soit congénitales, soit acquises.

Check only those questions to which you answer YES.
Cochez seulement les questions auxquelles vous répondez OUI.

Complaint
Symptômes
❑ I cannot urinate.

Je n'arrive pas à uriner.
- ❏ I have been unable to urinate for _____ minutes/hours/days.
  Je n'ai pas réussi à uriner depuis _____ minutes/heures/jours.
- ❏ I have pain in my right/left/both flank(s). (Refer to Anatomic Diagrams)
  J'ai mal au côté droit/gauche/aux deux côtés. (Voir les diagrammes anatomique)

Associated symptoms and history
Symptômes associés et informations complémentaires
- ❏ I have pain above my pubic bone. (Show the Groin Diagrams)
  J'ai mal au-dessus de l'os pubien. (Montrer les diagrammes de l'aine)
- ❏ I have pain in the right/left/both testicle(s).
  J'ai mal au testicule droit/gauche/aux deux testicules.
- ❏ I have pain in the right/left/both side(s) of my vagina.
  J'ai mal au côté droit/gauche/aux deux côtés du vagin.
- ❏ I have been drinking a lot of non-alcoholic beverages lately.
  Je consomme beaucoup de boissons non-alcolisées depuis quelque temps.
- ❏ I have been drinking a lot of alcoholic beverages lately.
  Je consomme beaucoup de boissons alcolisées depuis quelque temps.
- ❏ I have had this problem in the past. (Refer to Medical History)
  J'ai déjà eu ce problème. (Voir antécédents médicaux)
- ❏ I have a history of kidney stones.
  J'ai déjà eu des calculs dans les reins.
- ❏ I have a history of prostate cancer.
  J'ai déjà eu un cancer de la prostate.
- ❏ I have been taking a new medication. (Show the new medication and list of any previous medications.)
  Je prends un nouveau médicament. (Montrer le nouveau médicament ainsi que la liste de tous les anciens medicaments.)
- ❏ I have been taking this new medication for the past _____ days.
  Je prends ce nouveau médicament depuis _____ jours.

Vaginal Bleeding

Vaginal bleeding may be normal or abnormal. The following will be useful in providing pertinent information to your physician regarding this complaint.

Les saignements vaginaux

Les saignements vaginaux peuvent être normaux ou anormaux. Les questions ci-dessous seront utiles pour fournir à votre médecin des informations importantes sur ce dont vous souffrez.

Check only those questions to which you answer YES.
Cochez seulement les questions auxquelles vous répondez OUI.

Complaint
Symptômes
❑ I am having bleeding from my vagina.
　J'ai des saignements vaginaux.
❑ This has been occurring for the past _____ days/weeks.
　Cela se produit depuis _____ jours/semaines.
❑ I have a fever. (Refer to Temperature Scale)
　J'ai de la fièvre. (Voir l'échelle de température)

Associated symptoms and history
Symptômes associés et informations complémentaires
❑ The bleeding is intermittent.
　Les saignements sont intermittents.
❑ The bleeding is constant.
　Les saignements sont constants.
❑ I have passed tissue and blood.
　J'urine du sang et des particules solides.
❑ I have used _____ sanitary pads today.
　J'ai utilisé _____ serviettes hygiéniques aujourdhui.
❑ I have abdominal pain. (Refer to Abdominal Pain Section)
　J'ai une douleur abdominale. (Voir la section douleur abdominale)
❑ The pain is:
　La douleur est:
　　❑ constant.

constante.

❏ intermittent.

intermitente.

❏ remains in one location.

reste très localisée.

❏ goes to another location here: (Demonstrate)

se propage à cet endroit-ci: (Démontrer)

❏ I have nausea.

J'ai des nausées.

❏ I have diarrhea.

J'ai la diarrhée.

❏ I feel lightheaded.

J'ai la tête qui tourne.

❏ I have passed out.

Je me suis évanouie.

❏ I have a vaginal discharge.

J'ai des pertes vaginales.

❏ The vaginal discharge is:

Les pertes vaginales sont:

  ❏ yellow.

  jaunes.

  ❏ brown.

  marron.

  ❏ white.

  blanches.

❏ I urinate frequently.

J'urine fréquemment.

❏ I have pain when I urinate.

Cela me fait mal quand j'urine.

❏ I urinate in small volumes.

J'urine en petites quantités.

❏ I urinate at night.

J'urine la nuit.

❏ I have pain in my back. (Refer to Back Diagram)

J'ai mal au dos. (Voir le diagramme du dos)

❑ My last menstrual period was:
  Mes dernières règles étaient :
    ❑ light.
      peu abondantes.
    ❑ heavy.
      abondantes.
    ❑ normal.
      normales.
❑ My menstrual periods are regular.
  Mes règles sont régulières.
❑ I have a menstrual period monthly.
  J'ai mes règles chaque mois.
❑ I may be pregnant.
  Je suis peut-être enceinte.
❑ I am not pregnant.

  Je ne suis pas enceinte.
❑ I have been pregnant _____ times.
  J'ai déjà été enceinte _____ fois.
❑ I have had _____ deliveries.
  J'ai déjà accouché _____ fois.
❑ I have had _____ premature deliveries.
  J'ai déjà accouché prématurément _____ fois.
❑ I have had _____ miscarriages.
  J'ai déjà fait _____ fausses-couches.
❑ I have had an ectopic pregnancy.
  J'ai déjà eu une grossesse extra-utérine.
❑ I have had a sexually transmitted disease (STD) in the past. This
  was:
  J'ai déjà eu une maladie sexuellement transmissible (MST).
  C'était:
    ❑ gonorrhea.
      une blennorragie.
    ❑ syphilis.
      une syphilis.
    ❑ pelvic inflammatory disease.

une maladie inflammatoire pelvienne.
- ❏ herpes.

  un herpes.
- ❏ I don't know what STD I had.

  Je ne sais pas quelle MST j'ai eue.
- ❏ I recently had sexual intercourse.

  J'ai récemment eu des relations sexuelles.
- ❏ I/we use condoms.

  J'utilise/nous utilisons des préservatifs.
- ❏ I use an intrauterine device.

  J'utilise un dispositif intra-utérin.
- ❏ I use birth control pills.

  Je prends la pilule.
- ❏ I do not use any form of contraception.

  Je n'utilise aucune forme de contraception.
- ❏ I recently had trauma to my abdomen. (Demonstrate)

  J'ai récemment eu un traumatisme à l'abdomen. (Démontrer)

Pregnancy/Labor

Pregnancy may be complicated by recurrent nausea, vomiting, or abdominal pain. The following is extremely limited. If you are traveling while pregnant, bring all your medical records. These can be invaluable to your health care.

Labor can occur at full term or prematurely.

The following will be useful in providing pertinent information to your physician regarding these complaints.

La grossesse/l'accouchement

Une grossesse peut entraîner des complications sous forme de nausées, de douleurs abdominales et de vomissements récurrents. Les questions ci-dessous sont très succintes. Si vous voyagez enceinte, apportez avec vous votre dossier médical. Ces informations peuvent d'être d'une importance capitale pour votre santé.

L'accouchement peut avoir lieu à terme ou prématurément.

Les questions ci-dessous seront utiles pour fournir à votre médecin des informations importantes sur ce dont vous souffrez.

Complaint

Symptômes

❏ I have been vomiting for _____ minutes/hours/days. (Refer to the Vomiting Section)

Je vomis depuis _____ minutes/heures/jours. (Voir section vomissements)

❏ I have been nauseated for _____ minutes/hours/days. (Refer to the Nausea Section)

J'ai la nausée depuis _____ minutes/heures/jours. (Voir section nausée)

❏ I have had abdominal pain for _____ minutes/hours/days. (Refer to the Abdominal Pain Section)

Je ressens une douleur abdominale depuis _____ minutes/heures/jours. (Voir la section douleur abdominale)

❏ I have a fever. (Refer to Temperature Scale)

J'ai de la fièvre. (Voir l'échelle de température)

❏ I am _____ weeks pregnant.

Je suis enceinte de _____ semaines.

I am in labor.

Je suis en travail.

❏ The labor pains started _____ minutes/hours/days ago.

Les contractions ont débuté il y a _____ minutes/heures/jours.

❏ I am having contractions.

J'ai des contractions.

❏ The contractions occur every _____ minutes.

J'ai des contractions toutes les _____ minutes.

❏ The contractions last _____ minutes.

Ces contractions durent _____ minutes.

Associated symptoms and history

Symptômes associés et informations complémentaires

❏ My water has broken.

J'ai perdu les eaux.

❏ The color of the water was:

La couleur de l'eau était:

❏ clear.
  clair.
❏ yellow.
  jaune.
❏ red.
  rouge.
❏ My water broke at _____ AM/PM.
  J'ai perdu les eaux à _____ heures du matin/de l'après-midi/du
  soir.
❏ I am due on _____.
  L'accouchement est prévu pour le _____.
❏ I have had _____ full term pregnancies.
  J'ai déjà accouché à terme _____ fois.
❏ I have had _____ premature pregnancies.
  J'ai déjà accouché prématurément _____ fois.
❏ I have had _____ Caesarian sections.
  J'ai déjà accouché par césarienne _____ fois.
❏ I have had _____ miscarriages.
  J'ai déjà fait _____ fausses-couches.
❏ I have had _____ abortions.
  Je me suis déjà fait avorter _____ fois.
❏ I have had an episiotomy in the past.
  J'ai déjà subi une épisiotomie.
❏ I have had spinal analgesia in the past.
  J'ai déjà eu des péridurales.
❏ I have eclampsia.
  Je fais des crises d'éclampsie.
❏ I have had eclampsia with previous pregnancies.
  J'ai déjà fait des crises d'éclampsie lors de grossesses
  précédentes.
❏ I have hypertension.
  Je fais de l'hypertension.
❏ I have diabetes.
  J'ai du diabète.
❏ I have been healthy during my pregnancy.
  Je suis en bonne santé depuis le début de de ma grossesse.

❏ I have had premature labor with previous pregnancies. Medications were used to control this problem.

J'ai déjà eu des contractions prématurées lors de grossesses précédentes. On m'a prescrit des médicaments pour résoudre ce problème.

❏ I have had ectopic pregnancies in the past.

J'ai déjà eu des grossesses extra-utérines.

❏ I am _____ cm dilated.

J'avais le col dilaté de _____ cms.

❏ I have had heavy bleeding after previous deliveries.

J'ai déjà eu des saignements abondants à la suite d'accouchements précédents.

❏ I have used recreational drugs during this pregnancy.

J'ai continué à prendre des drogues douces pendant cette grossesse.

❏ I have used tobacco during this pregnancy.

J'ai continué à fumer du tabac pendant cette grossesse.

❏ I have used alcohol during this pregnancy.

J'ai continué à boire de l'alcool pendant cette grossesse.

❏ I have a bleeding disorder. (Refer to Medical History Section)

J'ai des saignements anormaux. (Voir la section antécédents médicaux)

EXTREMITIES
LES EXTRÉMITÉS

Joint Pain

Joint inflammation may occur acutely or develop over a long period of time. Joint pain may develop in association with a variety of other systemic disorders. For example, it may accompany sexually transmitted diseases. This section covers joint pain and other pertinent conditions relating to joint pain abnormalities. Evaluation of the joint includes the history, examination of the joint and other organ systems, and x-rays of the joint. It may also involve a joint tap which is the placement of a sterile needle into the joint space to allow examination of the joint fluid.

Pay particular attention to the following aspects of joint pain:
- Is there one joint in particular that is afflicted or are there multiple joints involved?
- Did the pain begin acutely or has it developed over a longer period of time?
- Has there been recent trauma to the area around the affected joint?
- Has there been any disruption of the skin integrity near the joint?

Les douleurs articulaires

Les inflammations articulaires peuvent apparaître soudainement ou se développer sur une longue période de temps. Les douleurs articulaires peuvent se développer conjointement avec toutes sortes d'autres troubles généralisés. Par exemple, des douleurs articulaires peuvent accompagner des maladies sexuellement transmissibles. La section ci-dessous couvre les douleurs articulaires ainsi que d'autres problèmes importants liés à des douleurs articulaires anormales. Le diagnostic concernant l'articulation comprendra les antécédents médicaux, l'examen de l'articulation et d'autres organes, des radioscopies de l'articulation et éventuellement une ponction articulaire (effectuée à l'aide d'une aiguille stérile que l'on place dans l'espace articulaire pour examiner le fluide articulaire).

Considérez attentivement les aspects suivants des douleurs articulaires:

• Y a-t-il seulement une articulation qui est affectée, ou de multiples articulations?
• La douleur articulaire est-elle apparue soudainement ou s'est-elle développée sur une plus longue période de temps?
• La zone qui entoure l'articulation affectée a-t-elle récemment fait l'objet d'un traumatisme?
• L'intégrité de la peau près de l'articulation a-t-elle été affectée?

Check only those questions to which you answer YES.
Cochez seulement les questions auxquelles vous répondez OUI.

Complaint
Symptômes
❑ I am having pain in my joints. (Refer to Diagrams)
　J'ai mal aux articulations. (Voir les diagrammes)
❑ I am having pain in many joints.
　J'ai mal à de nombreuses articulations.
❑ The pain is present on both sides of my body.
　J'ai mal des deux côtés du corps.
❑ This problem has been present for _____ hours/days/weeks.
　J'ai ce problème depuis _____ heures/jours/semaines.
❑ I have a fever. (Refer to Temperature Scale)
　J'ai de la fièvre. (Voir l'échelle de température)

Associated symptoms and history
Symptômes associés et informations complémentaires
❑ I have injured this joint in the past.
　Je me suis déjà fait mal à cette articulation.
❑ I have fractured this joint in the past.
　Je me suis déjà fracturé cette articulation.
❑ I have sprained this joint in the past.
　Je me suis déjà foulé cette articulation.
❑ I have had surgery on this joint in the past.
　Je me suis déjà fait opérer de cette articulation.
❑ I have used intravenous drugs recently.
　J'ai récemment pris des médicaments par intraveineuse.
❑ The pain started quickly.

La douleur a débuté très vite.
- ❏ I have a rash here. (Show)
  J'ai de l'urticaire à cet endroit-ci. (Montrer)
- ❏ I have aches and pains in my muscles.
  J'ai des douleurs et des courbatures dans les muscles.
- ❏ The pain is like a burning sensation.
  Je ressens comme une brûlure.
- ❏ I have numbness in the joint and in the area around the joint.
  Je n'ai plus de sensations dans cette articulation ni dans la zone tout autour.
- ❏ The joint(s) are stiff in the morning when I awake.
  Cette/Ces articulation(s) est/sont engourdie(s) le matin quand je me réveille.
- ❏ After about an hour, the pain has markedly improved.
  Au bout d'une heure environ, le douleur s'est amplifiée de façon notable.
- ❏ The pain is made worse by using the joint.
  La douleur s'accentue si je me sers de cette articulation.
- ❏ The pain is better when I rest the joint.
  La douleur s'atténue si je ne me sers pas de cette articulation.
- ❏ The pain is worse when I bear weight on the joint.
  La douleur s'accentue si j'appuie sur l'articulation.
- ❏ I have had similar pain in the past.
  J'ai déjà eu mal comme cela.
- ❏ This is the first time I have had this pain.
  C'est la première fois que j'ai mal commme cela.
- ❏ I have had pain like this in other joints.
  J'ai déjà eu mal comme cela à d'autres articulations.
- ❏ I have lost weight. I've lost _____ pounds over the last _____ weeks/months. (2.2 pounds = 1 kilogram)
  J'ai perdu du poids. J'ai perdu _____ kilos pendant les _____ dernières semaines/derniers mois.
- ❏ I have fatigue and malaise.
  Je suis fatigué(e) et j'ai des malaises.
- ❏ I have weakness in the area around the joint.
  La zone qui entoure l'articulation est toute molle.

❏ The pain is constant.

    J'ai mal en permanence.

❏ The pain is worse at night.

    La douleur s'amplifie la nuit.

❏ I have bumps here. (Show)

    J'ai des déformations nodales là. (Montrer)

❏ I have been losing my hair.

    Je perds mes cheveux.

❏ I have ulcers in my mouth.

    J'ai des ulcères dans la bouche.

❏ I have ulcers in my nose.

    J'ai des ulcères dans le nez.

❏ I have dry eyes and mouth.

    J'ai la bouche et les yeux secs.

❏ I have had eye problems recently.

    J'ai eu des problèmes à l'œil récemment.

❏ I have chest pain that becomes worse when I take a deep breath.

    J'ai une douleur à la poitrine qui s'amplifie quand j'inspire
      profondément.

❏ My fingers turn white when they are cold.

    Mes doigts deviennent tout blancs quand ils sont froids.

❏ My fingers are painful when they are cold.

    Mes doigts me font mal quand ils sont froids.

❏ I have nausea. (Refer to Nausea Section)

    J'ai la nausée. (Voir section nausée)

❏ I have been vomiting. (Refer to Vomiting Section.)

    J'ai des vomissements. (Voir section vomissements)

❏ I have diarrhea. (Refer to Diarrhea Section.)

    J'ai la diarrhée. (Voir section diarrhée)

❏ I have a stiff neck.

    J'ai une raideur dans la nuque.

❏ I have a headache. (Refer to Headache Section)

    J'ai mal à la tête. (Voir la section des maux de tête.)

❏ I am sexually active.

    J'ai une vie sexuelle.

❏ I have a discharge from my penis. (Refer to Sexually Transmitted

Diseases Section)

J'ai un écoulement du pénis. (Voir les maladies transmises sexuellement.)

❏ I have a discharge from my vagina. (Refer to Sexually Transmitted Diseases Section)

J'ai des pertes vaginales. (Voir les maladies transmises sexuellement)

❏ I have a discharge from my rectum.

J'ai des pertes rectales.

❏ I have had sexual relations with a new partner recently.

J'ai eu des rapports sexuels avec un nouveau partenaire/une nouvelle partenaire récemment.

❏ I have a joint replacement. (Show the joint)

J'ai une prothèse articulaire. (Montrez l'articulation concernée)

❏ I have HIV infection. I am seropositve.

J'ai une infection par le virus HIV. Je suis séropositif.

❏ I have AIDS.

J'ai le sida.

❏ The pain started quickly and peaked several hours later.

La douleur a débuté très vite et a culminé plusieurs heures après.

❏ I have pain when I move the joint.

J'ai mal quand je bouge les articulations.

❏ I have pain when I do not move the joint.

J'ai mal quand je ne bouge pas les articulations.

❏ The joint(s) is red/swollen/both.

J'ai les articulations toute rouges/gonflées/les deux.

❏ I have traveled to _____ (city/country).

Je suis allé(e) à/en (aux) _____ (ville/pays).

❏ I have been in the northeastern United States. (Note to healthcare provider: consider Lyme Disease)

Je suis allé(e) dans le nord-est des Etats-Unis (Note au praticien de santé: penser à la maladie de Lyme)

❏ I have rheumatoid arthritis.

J'ai une arthrite rhumatoïde.

❏ I have osteoarthritis.

J'ai une ostéoarthrite.

❑ I have sarcoidosis.
  J'ai une sarcoïdose.
❑ I have systemic lupus erythematosis.
  J'ai un lupus erythemateux aigu disséminé.
❑ I have Crohn's disease
  J'ai la maladie de Crohn.
❑ I have ulcerative colitis.
  J'ai une colite ulcérative.
❑ I have had my spleen removed.
  Je me suis fait enlever la rate.
❑ I have a large spleen.
  J'ai une grosse rate.
❑ I have leukemia.
  J'ai une leucémie.
❑ I have fibromyalgia.
  J'ai une fibromyalgie.
❑ I have taken _____ aspirin tablets over the past 24 hours. I have
  done this for the last _____ days/weeks.
  J'ai pris de l'aspirine. J'ai pris _____ comprimés durant les 24
  heures qui viennent de s'écouler. Je fais cela depuis _____
  jours/semaines.
❑ I have taken _____ acetaminophen tablets over the past 24 hours.
  I have done this for the last _____ days/weeks.
  J'ai pris. J'ai pris _____ comprimés de l'acétaminophène durant
  les 24 heures qui viennent de s'écouler. Je fais cela depuis
  _____jours/semaines.
❑ I have taken my usual medications. (Refer to Medications Section)
  J'ai pris mes médicaments habituels. (Voir section médicaments)

Back Pain
Back pain may be acute or a recurring problem. The following questions will assist you in relating pertinent information to your physician regarding this medical problem.

Les douleurs dorsales
Les douleurs dorsales peuvent être un problème aigu ou un problème
récurrent. Les questions suivantes vous aideront à communiquer des

informations importantes à votre médecin concernant ce problème médical.

Check only those questions to which you answer YES.
Cochez seulement les questions auxquelles vous répondez OUI.

Complaint
Symptômes
❏ I have back pain. (Refer to Back Diagrams)
　J'ai mal au dos. (Voir les diagrammes du dos.)
❏ The problem has been present for ＿＿＿ hours/days/weeks.
　J'ai ce problème depuis ＿＿＿ heures/jours/semaines.

Associated symptoms and history
Symptômes associés et informations complémentaires
❏ I have pain on the right/left/both sides.
　J'ai mal à droite/à gauche/des deux côtés.
❏ I have problems with low back pain. Please see my medical history.
　J'ai souvent mal dans le bas du dos. Veuillez consulter mes
　　antécédents médicaux.
❏ The pain started all of a sudden.
　La douleur a débuté soudainement.
❏ The pain started gradually.
　La douleur a débuté progressivement.
❏ The pain is always present.
　J'ai mal en permanence.
❏ The pain comes and goes.
　J'ai mal de façon intermittente.
❏ The pain is very brief.
　La douleur est très brève.
❏ The pain is sharp like a knife.
　La douleur est intense, comme si on me donnait un coup de
　　couteau.
❏ The pain is a dull aching sensation.
　La douleur est soured.
❏ The pain started after I lifted a heavy object.
　J'ai commencé à avoir mal après avoir soulevé un objet lourd.

❑ The pain started after an injury.
   J'ai commencé à avoir mal après m'être blessé(e).
❑ The injury occurred _____ hours/days/weeks ago.
   Je me suis blessé(e) il y a _____ heures/jours/semaines.
❑ I cannot recall having injured my back recently.
   Je ne me souviens pas de m'être fait mal au dos récemment.
❑ The pain stays in my back.
   La douleur reste dans le dos.
❑ The pain shoots down into the back of my legs on the
   right/left/both side(s).
   Le douleur s'étend à l'arrière de mes jambes du côté
   droit/gauche/des deux côtés.
❑ The pain shoots into my abdomen. (Demonstrate)
   Le douleur s'étend à l'abdomen. (Démontrer)
❑ The pain shoots into my testicles/vagina on the right/left/both
   side(s).
   La douleur s'étend aux testicules/ au vagin au côté
   droit/gauche/des deux côtés.
❑ I have a fever. (Refer to Temperature Scale)
   J'ai de la fièvre. (Voir l'échelle de température)
❑ I have been vomiting. (Refer to Vomiting Section)
   J'ai des vomissements. (Voir section vomissements)
❑ I have difficulty urinating. (Refer to Urinary Tract Section)
   J'ai du mal à uriner. (Voir section voies urinaires)
❑ I have seen red blood in my urine. (Refer to Kidney Section)
   J'ai constaté la présence de sang rouge dans mes urines. (Voir la
   section des reins.)
❑ I have had kidney stones in the past.
   J'ai déjà eu des calculs dans les reins.
❑ I have a cough. (Refer to Cough Section.)
   Je tousse. (Voir section toux)
❑ The pain is worse when I cough or breathe deeply. (Refer to
   Pulmonary Section)
   La douleur s'accentue quand je tousse ou respire profondément.
   (Voir section pulmonaire)

Skin Infection

This section is designed to report information about skin infections (cellulitis). Most skin infections are red, tender, and warm. They are usually bacterial and not viral in nature. The infection may have been preceded by a break in the skin. Underlying diseases such as diabetes and peripheral vasculature insufficiency may predispose patients to the development of skin infections. A history of trauma is also important. The location of the infection is helpful for the physician to assess the potential causes of the infection. Certain bacteria tend to commonly infect certain body areas.

Les infections cutanées

Cette section a été conçue pour fournir des renseignements sur les infections cutanées (cellulites). La peau, dans la plupart des cas d'infections cutanées, est rouge, sensible et chaude. L'infection est généralement bactérielle et non virale. Elle peut être précédée d'une coupure à la peau. Des maladies sous-jacentes telles que le diabète et l'insuffisance vasculaire périphérique peuvent prédisposer les patients à développer des infections cutanées. Il est aussi important de connaître les antécédents du patient en matière de traumatisme. Il est utile pour le médecin de savoir où se situe l'infection pour en déterminer les causes éventuelles. Certain bactéries ont tendance très souvent à infecter certaines parties du corps.

Check only those questions to which you answer YES.
Cochez seulement les questions auxquelles vous répondez OUI.

Complaint
Symptômes
❏ I have a rash.
　 J'ai de l'urticaire.
❏ The rash began _____ hours/days ago.
　 L'urticaire a débuté il y a _____ heures/jours.
❏ I have a fever. (Refer to Temperature Scale)
　 J'ai de la fièvre. (Voir l'échelle de température)

Associated symptoms and history
Symptômes associés et informations complémentaires

❏ I have had trauma to the area recently. (Demonstrate)
   Je me suis récemment fait mal à cet endroit-là. (Démontrer)
❏ I have injected drugs (legal/illegal) recently.
   J e me suis récemment fait une injection de drogue
   (légale/illégale).
❏ I have diabetes mellitus.
   J'ai un diabète sucré.
❏ I had a sore throat recently.
   J'ai eu mal à la gorge récemment.
❏ I have had blood drawn recently.
   J'ai eu une prise de sang récemment.
❏ I have had a lymph node dissection. This was for:
   J'ai subi une dissection du nodule lymphatique à cause d'un :
      ❏ breast cancer.
         cancer du sein.
      ❏ malignant melanoma.
         mélanome malin.
      ❏ gynecologic cancer.
         cancer gynécologique.
❏ I have had the veins in my legs harvested for my heart operation.
   On a utilisé les veines de mes jambes pour m'opérer du cœur.
❏ I have been handling fish, meat, poultry lately.
   J'ai manipulé du poisson, de la viande et de la volaille
   récemment.
❏ I have been swimming in the ocean.
   Je me suis baigné(e) dans l'océan.
❏ I have been swimming in fresh water. (river, lake, etc.)
   Je me suis baigné(e) en eau douce. (fleuve, lac, etc.)
❏ I have been swimming in a pool.
   Je me suis baigné(e) en piscine.
❏ I have been bitten by a dog.
   J'ai été mordu(e) par un chien.
❏ I have been bitten by a cat.
   J'ai été mordu(e) par un chat.

TRAUMA
LES TRAUMATISMS

Eye Injury/Trauma

Eye injuries are usually the result of trauma. The trauma may be slight, such as from contact lens irritation or a corneal abrasion, or more overt like direct trauma to the head. The treatment of ocular injuries is directed at resolving the acute problem with respect to pain control and preservation of sight. The role of an ophthalmologist in ocular injuries is paramount to good care. If your physician has made a recommendation for follow-up with an ophthalmologist, it is extremely beneficial for you to heed this advice.

Routine treatments of ocular injuries include eye patches and topical antibiotics. Pain from ocular injuries can be quite severe, especially with a corneal abrasion. The initial treatment usually results in complete pain control. However, the pain is likely to return later. Continued use of the topical anesthetic used in this situation may actually impair corneal repair if used on a chronic basis. Be sure that you have discussed this with your physician. If the pain is severe, oral analgesics may be prescribed.

Les blessures à l'œil/les traumatismes de l'œil

Les blessures à l'œil proviennent généralement d'un traumatisme. Le traumatisme peut être léger, comme dans le cas d'une irritation due à une lentille de contact: abrasion cornéenne, ou plus important comme dans le cas d'un traumatisme direct à la tête. Le traitement des blessures oculaires vise à résoudre la crise aiguë tout en contrôlant la douleur et préservant la vue. Le rôle de l'ophtalmologiste dans le cas des blessures oculaires est essentiel pour être bien soigné. Si votre médecin vous a recommandé de vous faire suivre médicalement chez un ophtalmologiste, il est dans votre intérêt de suivre ce conseil.

Les traitements systématiques des blessures oculaires comprennent des caches pour les yeux et des antibiotiques ponctuels. La douleur provenant des blessures oculaires peut être très vive, particulièrement dans le cas d'une abrasion cornéenne. Le traitement initial a généralement pour effet de stopper complètement la douleur. Néanmoins, il se peut que la douleur réapparaisse plus tard. L'utilisation prolongée de l'anesthésique ponctuel utilisé dans cette situation particulière peut, en fait, compromettre la réparation de la cornée s'il est utilisé de façon chronique. Si la douleur est très importante, des analgésiques par voie buccale pourront également être prescrits.

Check only those questions to which you answer YES.
Cochez seulement les questions auxquelles vous répondez OUI.

Complaint
Symptômes

❑ I have an injury to my left/right/both eye(s).
Je me suis fait mal à l'œil gauche/droit/aux deux yeux.

❑ I have something in my eye. It is:
J'ai quelque chose dans l'œil. C'est:

❑ my contact lens (soft/hard/permeable).
ma lentille de contact (souple/dure/perméable à l'oxygène).

❑ an object: dirt/sand/metal/wood.
un corps étranger: une poussière/un grain de sable/un morceau de metal/de bois.

❑ liquid: chemical/gas/solvent/cleaner/other.
un produit liquide: produit chimique/gazeux/solvant detergent/autre.

❑ I do not think anything is in my eye.
Je ne pense pas avoir quoi que ce soit dans l'œil.

❑ I was struck in the eye with an object. It was:
J'ai reçu un coup à l'œil. Cela provenait:

❑ a blunt object.
d'un objet contondant.

❑ ball/hand/other.
d'un ballon/d'une main/autre.

❑ a sharp object.
d'un objet pointu.

❑ stick/knife/other.
d'un baton/d'un couteau/autre.

❑ My eyes(s) were burned.
Je me suis brûlé l'œil/les yeux.

❏ My vision is normal.
  Je vois normalement.
❏ My vision is not normal.
  Je ne vois pas normalement.
❏ I cannot keep my eye open.
  Je n'arrive pas à garder l'œil ouvert.
❏ I cannot see at all.
  Je ne vois rien du tout.
❏ I can see but my vision is:
  J'arrive à voir mais je vois:
    ❏ dim.
      mal.
    ❏ blurred.
      flou.

Associated symptoms and history
Symptômes associés et informations complémentaires
❏ I have pain. (Refer to Visual Pain Scale)
  J'ai mal. (Voir l'échelle de douleur)
❏ The pain is throbbing/dull/sharp/intermittent/constant. (Circle all
  that apply)
  La douleur est aiguë/sourde/intense/intermittente/
    constante. (Entourez la ou les bonne(s) réponse(s))
❏ I also have other injuries. (Show)
  Je me suis aussi fait mal ailleurs. (Montrer)
❏ I am nauseated.
  J'ai la nausée.
❏ I have a fever. (Refer to Temperature Scale)
  J'ai de la fièvre. (Voir l'échelle de température)
❏ I have washed the eye.
  Je me suis nettoyé l'œil.
❏ I have used eye drops. (Show eye drops)
  Je me suis mis des gouttes dans l'œil/les yeux. (Montrer les
    gouttes pour les yeux)
❏ I have tried to get an object out.
  J'ai essayé de retirer un corps étranger de mon œil.

❑ I have no prior eye problems.
  Je n'ai jamais eu de problèmes à l'œil/aux yeux.
❑ I wear glasses.
  Je porte des lunettes.
❑ I wear contact lenses.
  Je porte des lentilles de contact.
❑ I have:
  J'ai:
    ❑ cataracts.
      une cataracte.
    ❑ glaucoma.
      un glaucome.
❑ I use medications for my eyes. (Refer to Medication Section)
  Je prends des médicaments pour les yeux. (Voir section
  medicaments)

Nose Trauma
Please be sure that the first section regarding your medical history,
current medications, allergies, etc. has been filled out completely.

Les traumatismes du nez
Veuillez vous assurer d'avoir complété soigneusement la première
section concernant vos antécédents médicaux, vos traitements en
cours, et vos allergies, etc.

Check only those questions to which you answer YES.
Cochez seulement les questions auxquelles vous répondez OUI.

Complaint
Symptômes
❑ My nose is injured.
  Je me suis blessé(e) au nez.
❑ I was hit in the nose.
  On m'a frappé(e) au nez.
❑ I fell.
  Je suis tombé(e).
❑ This happened _____ minutes/hours/days ago.

Cela s'est produit il y a _____ minutes/heures/jours.

I have pain. (Refer to Visual Pain Scale)

J'ai mal (Voir l'échelle de douleur)

❑ The pain is:

La douleur est:

   ❑ throbbing.

     aiguë.

   ❑ dull.

     sourde.

   ❑ sharp.

     intense.

   ❑ intermittent.

     intermittente.

   ❑ constant.

     constante.

❑ I also injured my: (Refer to Head Diagram)

Je me suis aussi fait mal: (Voir les diagrammes de la tête)

   ❑ teeth.

     aux dents.

   ❑ jaw.

     a la mâchoire.

   ❑ eye or eyes.

     a l'œil ou aux yeux.

Head Injury/Concussion

A concussion results from a blow to the head. It is defined by an alteration in brain function. A minor blow may cause one to be "dazed" but not lose consciousness. Any more serious injury is associated with loss of consciousness for seconds to minutes. More serious injuries include bruising (contusion) of the brain or bleeding inside the skull. The skull may be broken but the resulting injury to the brain is usually more important. In the USA it is common to perform a CT scan of the brain for any head injury with loss of consciousness. This is not likely to be the practice in most other countries where observation for worsening injuries is used. The most sensitive test for brain injury is noting a change in personality. Pupil changes are not a good test for brain injury.

Les blessures à la tête/les commotions cérébrales

Une commotion cérébrale résulte d'un coup à la tête. Elle consiste en une altération des fonctions cérébrales. Un léger coup peut provoquer un étourdissement mais non une perte de conscience. Toute autre blessure sérieuse s'accompagne d'une perte de conscience, pendant quelques secondes ou quelques minutes. Il y a des blessures les plus graves comme les hématomes cérébraux ou les hémorragies cérébrales. La boîte crânienne peut être fracturée, mais la blessure au cerveau qui en résulte est généralement plus grave. Aux Etats-Unis, il est fréquent de procéder à un scanner du cerveau pour toute blessure à la tête ayant entraîné une perte de conscience. Ce ne sera certainement pas le cas dans la plupart des autres pays où l'on met les patients en observation pour voir si leurs blessures s'aggravent. Le test le plus sûr pour voir s'il y a eu une blessure au cerveau est de constater un changement de personnalité. Les changements constatés au niveau des pupilles ne représentent pas un bon test pour voir s'il y a une blessure au cerveau.

Check only those questions to which you answer YES.
Cochez seulement les questions auxquelles vous répondez OUI.

Complaint
Symptômes

❏ I have a head injury.
Je me suis blessé(e) à la tête.
❏ I fell down and struck my head.
Je suis tombé(e) et me suis cogné la tête.
❏ I fell ____ feet. (1 foot = 0.30 meters)
Je suis tombé(e) d'une hauteur de ____ centimètres/mètres.
❏ I was struck in the head.
On m'a frappé(e) à la tête.
❏ I was unconscious for ____ minutes.
Je suis resté(e) sans connaissance pendant ____ minutes.
❏ I was not unconscious.
Je n'ai pas perdu connaissance.
❏ I remember the injury.
Je me souviens de la façon dont je me suis blessé(e).

❏ I do not remember the injury.

Je ne me souviens pas de la façon dont je me suis blessé(e).

❏ I have a headache.

J'ai mal à la tête.

❏ I have pain. (Refer to Visual Pain Scale)

J'ai mal. (Voir l'échelle de douleur.)

❏ My vision is normal.

Je vois normalement.

❏ My vision is not normal.

Je ne vois pas normalement.

❏ I feel nauseated.

J'ai la nausée.

❏ I have vomited _____ times.

J'ai vomi _____ fois.

❏ I also have a laceration (cut).

Je me suis également coupé(e).

❏ I have neck pain. (Refer to Neck Pain and Injury Sections)

J'ai mal à la nuque. (Voir les sections blessures à la nuque)

❏ I am dizzy/I have balance problems.

J'ai des vertiges/j'ai des problèmes d'équilibre.

❏ I am lightheaded. I feel as if I may black out.

J'ai la tête qui tourne. J'ai l'impression que je vais m'évanouir.

❏ I have taken acetaminophen (Tylenol).

J'ai pris de l'acétaminophène (Tylenol).

❏ I have taken ibuprofen.

J'ai pris de l'ibuprofène.

❏ I have taken another medicine: _____.

J'ai pris un autre medicament: _____.

❏ I also have other injuries. (Show appropriate sections)

Je me suis aussi fait mal à d'autres endroits. (Préciser les zones concernées).

To be filled out by another person
A compléter par une autre personne

❏ He/she is confused.

Il/elle a l'esprit confus.

❏ He/she keeps repeating himself/herself.

Il/elle se répète.

❏ He/she is acting strange.

Il/elle se comporte bizarrement.

❏ He/she knows where he/she is.

Il/elle sait où il/elle est.

❏ He/she knows who he/she is.

Il/elle sait qui il/elle est.

❏ He/she knows the date.

Il/elle sait quel jour nous sommes.

Neck Injury

Neck injuries are very common and can be devastating. Motor vehicle crashes or falls cause most serious neck and spinal cord injuries. A neck can be broken without causing paralysis. One might be able to walk into a hospital with a broken neck. The most serious problems after neck injury are numbness or weakness in the arms or legs.

A cut to the neck can obviously be very serious and usually requires immediate attention. Non-traumatic neck pain is usually less serious. A disc problem (pinched nerve in the neck) can be quite painful but is more serious if it is causing loss of function in the arm(s).

Les blessures à la nuque

Les blessures à la nuque sont très courantes et peuvent avoir des effets dévastateurs. Les accidents de la circulation ou les chutes de moto sont la cause de la plupart des lésions médullaires graves au niveau cervical. On peut se casser la nuque sans que cela n'entraîne de paralysie. On peut se rendre soi-même à l'hôpital la nuque cassée. Les problèmes les plus graves qui peuvent résulter d'une blessure à la nuque sont l'absence de sensations ou les faiblesses que cette blessure peut provoquer dans les bras ou les jambes.

Une coupure au cou ou à la nuque peut être évidemment très grave et doit généralement être examinée immédiatement. Les douleurs à la nuque qui ne résultent pas d'un traumatisme sont généralement moins graves. Un problème discal (compression nerveuse dans la nuque) peut être très douloureux, mais il est plus grave s'il entraîne une perte de motricité des bras.

Check only those questions to which you answer YES.
Cochez seulement les questions auxquelles vous répondez OUI.

Complaint
Symptômes

❏ I have injured my neck.
   Je me suis fait mal à la nuque.

❏ I fell _____ feet. (1 foot = 0.30 meters)
   Je suis tombé(e) d'une hauteur de _____ centimètres/mètres.

❏ I twisted my neck.
   Je me suis tordu la nuque.

❏ I was hit on the neck.
   On m'a frappé(e) à la nuque.

❏ My neck hurts but I do not remember an injury.
   J'ai mal à la nuque mais je ne me souviens pas de m'être fait mal.

❏ My neck hurts in the back/front/left side/right side.
   J'ai mal à la nuque/au cou/au côté gauche de la nuque/au côté
   droit de la nuque.

❏ I have pain/numbness/weakness in my left arm/hands/fingers.
   J'ai mal/je n'ai plus de sensations/j'ai une faiblesse dans le bras
   gauche/mains/doigts.

❏ I have pain/numbness/weakness in my right arm/hands/fingers.
   J'ai mal/je n'ai plus de sensations/j'ai une faiblesse dans le bras
   droit/mains/doigts.

❏ I have pain/numbness/weakness in my left/right leg.
   J'ai mal à la jambe (gauche/droite)/je n'ai plus de sensations/j'ai
   une faiblesse dans la jambe gauche/droite.

❏ Indicate location of pain and numbness on the Anatomical
   Diagrams.
   Préciser l'endroit douloureux et l'endroit où il n'y a plus de
   sensations sur le diagramme externe du corps.

❏ I cannot move my left/right/hand/arm/leg normally.
   Je ne peux pas bouger normalement la main/le bras/la
   jambe/gauche/droit(e)

❏ This occurred _____ minutes/hours/days ago).
   Cela s'est produit il y a _____ minutes/heures/jours.

❏ I have pain. (Refer to Visual Pain Scale)

J'ai mal. (Voir l'échelle de douleur.)

❏ My upper/lower back also hurts.

J'ai également mal dans le haut/dans le bas du dos.

❏ My head hurts.

J'ai mal à la tête.

❏ I also have other injuries. (Show)

J'ai également mal à d'autres endroits. (Montrer)

❏ I have taken acetaminophen (Tylenol).

J'ai pris de l'acétaminophène (Tylenol).

❏ I have taken ibuprofen.

J'ai pris de l'ibuprofène.

❏ I have taken other medicine(s): _____.

J'ai pris d'autres medicaments: _____.

❏ I have had a previous neck injury.

Je me fais souvent mal à la nuque.

❏ I have had a previous disk injury.

J'ai déjà eu une lésion discale.

❏ I have had a previous bone injury.

J'ai déjà eu une lésion osseuse.

❏ I have arthritis in my neck.

J'ai de l'arthrite à la nuque.

❏ My injury was similar to this.

Ma blessure précédente était semblable à celle-ci.

❏ This is different from my previous injury.

Cette blessure-ci est différente de la précédente.

Leg/Ankle/Foot Injury
(sprains, muscle injury, broken bones)

A sprain is an injury to a ligament, a stretch or a tear. Ligaments connect bones together. A strain is an injury to a muscle or a tendon. Tendons connect muscles to bones. A contusion is a bruise to the muscle. A break and a fracture are the same thing: an injury to the bone.

You cannot tell if you have a fracture by the ability to move. You might be able to walk on a broken leg or ankle. If your injury seems mild you should be able to safely wait several days to see if it gets better. Serious injuries, ones that need immediate surgery or casting, are usually quite obvious.

Les blessures aux jambe/cheville/pied
(entorses, blessures musculaires, fractures)

Une entorse est une blessure à un ligament, étirement ou déchirure. Les ligaments relient les os les uns aux autres. Un claquage musculaire ou une tendinite sont des blessures à un muscle ou à un tendon. Les tendons relient les muscles aux os. Une contusion est un hématome au muscle. Une cassure et une fracture représentent la même chose: une lésion à l'os.

Vous ne pouvez pas juger si vous avez une fracture ou non par votre capacité à bouger. Il se peut même que vous puissiez marcher avec une cheville cassée. Si votre blessure vous semble mineure, vous devriez être en mesure d'attendre plusieurs jours, sans prendre de risques, pour voir si elle s'améliore. Il est généralement très facile de reconnaître les blessures graves, celles qui requièrent une opération ou un plâtrage immédiat.

Check only those questions to which you answer YES.
Cochez seulement les questions auxquelles vous répondez OUI.

Complaint
Symptômes
❑ I have injured my:
    Je me suis fait mal:
        ❑ upper leg.
          à la cuisse.
        ❑ lower leg.
          à la jambe.
        ❑ ankle.
          à la cheville.
        ❑ foot.

au pied.
- ❏ I think it is:
  Je pense qu'il/elle est:
  - ❏ broken.
    cassé(e).
  - ❏ sprained.
    foulé(e).
  - ❏ bruised.
    contusionné(e).
- ❏ The problem started _____ minutes/hours/days ago.
  Le problème a débuté il y a _____ minutes/heures/jours.
- ❏ I fell down.
  Je suis tombé(e).
- ❏ I fell _____ feet. (1 foot = 0.30 meters)
  Je suis tombé(e) d'une hauteur de _____ centimètres/mètres.
- ❏ I twisted my ankle.
  Je me suis tordu la cheville.
- ❏ I can walk.
  Je peux marcher.
- ❏ I cannot walk.
  Je ne peux pas marcher.
- ❏ I can move my knee.
  Je peux bouger le genou.
- ❏ I cannot move my knee.
  Je ne peux pas bouger le genou.
- ❏ I can move my ankle.
  Je peux bouger la cheville.
- ❏ I cannot move my ankle.
  Je ne peux pas bouger la cheville.
- ❏ It hurts here: (Demonstrate)
  J'ai mal là: (Démontrer)
- ❏ I have a numb area here: (Demonstrate)
  Je n'ai plus de sensations à cet endroit-là: (Démontrer)
- ❏ I also have a cut. (Demonstrate)
  Je me suis aussi coupé(e). (Démontrer)

❏ I injured this same extremity _____ months ago.

Je me suis déjà fait mal à cette extrémité il y a _____ mois.

❏ I have had surgery on this extremity.

J'ai déjà subi une opération de cette extrémité.

❏ I last ate or drank _____ hours ago.

J'ai mangé ou bu pour la dernière fois il y a _____ heures.

❏ I have taken acetaminophen (Tylenol).

J'ai pris de l'acétaminophène (Tylénol).

❏ I have taken ibuprofen.

J'ai pris de l'ibuprofène.

❏ I have taken another medicine: _____.

J'ai pris un autre medicament: _____.

Knee Injury
(sprains, muscle injury, broken bones)

The knee is a frequently injured joint. Very few knee injuries require immediate surgery. Even if surgery were required you could travel home. The knee can be sprained (a stretched or torn ligament). There are four main ligaments in the knee: medial and lateral collateral ligaments, anterior and posterior cruciate ligaments (the big ones). The cartilage or meniscus which is inside the knee joint can be torn, causing pain and swelling. The knee is not often broken. This requires a lot of force such as a very bad fall or an auto crash. The knee rarely dislocates but the knee cap can dislocate rather easily.

Les blessures au genou
(entorses, blessures musculaires, fractures)

Le genou est une articulation qui se blesse fréquemment. Très peu de blessures du genou requièrent une opération immédiate. Et même si une opération s'imposait, vous pourriez quand même rentrer chez vous. Le genou peut être foulé en raison d'un ligament étiré ou déchiré. Il y a 4 ligaments principaux dans le genou : les ligaments collatéraux médial et latéral, et les ligaments croisés antérieur et postérieur (les plus gros). Le cartilage ou ménisque qui se trouve à l'intérieur de l'articulation du genou peut se déchirer, provoquant des douleurs et faisant enfler le genou. Le genou ne se casse pas souvent. Cela demande beaucoup de force, comme une énorme chute ou un accident de voiture. De la même façon, le genou se luxe rarement (sauf, encore une fois, dans un accident de voiture), mais la rotule, en revanche, peut se luxer assez facilement.

Check only those questions to which you answer YES.
Cochez seulement les questions auxquelles vous répondez OUI.

Complaint
Symptômes
❏ I have injured my right knee.
    Je me suis fait mal au genou droit.
❏ I have injured my left knee.
    Je me suis fait mal au genou gauche.
❏ The problem started _____ minutes/hours/days ago.
    Le problème a débuté il y a _____ minutes/heures/jours.
❏ I have pain. (Refer to Visual Pain Scale)
    J'ai mal. (Voir l'échelle de douleur)
❏ It hurts in the:
    J'ai mal:
    ❏ front.
       sur le devant.
    ❏ back.
       a l'arrière.
    ❏ inside.
       a l'intérieur.
    ❏ outside.
       a l'extérieur.
❏ My patella (kneecap) hurts.
    J'ai mal à la rotule.
❏ It is swollen.
    Mon genou est enflé.
❏ It has been swollen for _____ minutes/hours/days.
    Mon genou est enflé depuis _____ minutes/heures/jours.
❏ I can walk on it.
    Je peux marcher.

❏ It hurts when I walk on it.
  Mon genou me fait mal quand je marche.
❏ It does not hurt when I walk on it.
  Mon genou ne me fait pas mal quand je marche.
❏ It popped when I hurt it.
  Mon genou s'est déboîté quand je me suis fait mal.
❏ It pops when I walk on it.
  Mon genou se déboîte quand je marche.
❏ It gives out when I walk on it.
  Mon genou flanche quand je marche.
❏ I cannot bend my knee.
  Je ne peux pas plier le genou.
❏ I cannot straighten my knee.
  Je ne peux pas étendre le genou.
❏ My leg is numb below the knee.
  Je n'ai plus de sensations dans la jambe au-dessous du genou.
❏ Part of my leg is numb. (Demonstrate)
  Je n'ai plus de sensations dans une partie de la jambe.
   (Démontrer)
❏ I have other injuries (Demonstrate)
  J'ai mal à d'autres endroits du corps. (Démontrer)
❏ I have had a previous injury to this knee.
  Je me suis déjà fait mal à ce genou.
❏ This injury seems the same.
  Cette blessure semble être la même.
❏ This injury seems different.
  Cette blessure semble être différente.
❏ I have had surgery on this knee.
  J'ai déjà subi une opération de ce genou.
❏ I have had a surgical repair of my anterior cruciate ligament.
  J'ai déjà subi une opération du ligament croisé antérieur.
❏ I have had a surgical repair of my posterior cruciate ligament.
  J'ai déjà subi une opération du ligament croisé postérieur.
❏ I have had arthroscopic surgery on this knee.
  J'ai déjà subi une athroscopie du genou.

Shoulder Injury

Shoulder injuries are usually caused by a fall onto the arm or shoulder. If you fall directly on the shoulder it is more likely to break the shoulder (humerus bone), separate the acromioclavicular joint, or break the clavicle. A fall onto an arm may tear the shoulder muscles and ligaments or dislocate the shoulder. Pain without trauma may be caused by bursitis (an inflammation of the lubricating sac) or a pinched nerve.

Les blessures à l'épaule

Les blessures à l'épaule sont généralement causées par une chute sur le bras ou l'épaule. Si vous tombez directement sur l'épaule, cela risque de casser l'épaule (l'humérus), de séparer l'articulation acromio-claviculaire ou de casser la clavicule. Une chute sur un bras peut entraîner une déchirure des muscles et des ligaments de l'épaule ou une luxation de l'épaule. Une douleur sans traumatisme peut avoir été causée par une bursite, c'est-à-dire une inflammation du liquide synovial ou une compression nerveuse.

Check only those questions to which you answer YES.
Cochez seulement les questions auxquelles vous répondez OUI.

Complaint
Symptômes
❏ I have injured my shoulder.
   Je me suis fait mal à l'épaule.
❏ My shoulder hurts but I have not injured it.
   J'ai mal à l'épaule mais je ne me suis pas blessé(e) à l'épaule.
❏ I think it is:
   Je pense qu'elle est:
   ❏ broken.
      cassée.
   ❏ sprained.
      foulée.
   ❏ bruised.
      contusionnée.
❏ The problem started minutes/hours/days ago.
   Le problème a débuté il y a _____ minutes/heures/jours.

❏ I fell down.
   Je suis tombé(e).
❏ I fell _____ feet. (1 foot = 0.30 meters)
   Je suis tombé(e) d'une hauteur de _____ centimètres/mètres.
❏ My arm was against my side when I fell.
   J'avais le bras le long du corps quand je suis tombé(e).
❏ My arm was above my head when I fell.
   J'avais le bras levé au-dessus de la tête quand je suis tombé(e).
❏ I can move my shoulder.
   Je peux bouger l'épaule.
❏ I cannot move my shoulder.
   Je ne peux pas bouger l'épaule.
❏ My hand and arm feel normal.
   J'ai des sensations normales dans la main et dans le bras.
❏ Part of my hand or arm feels asleep is numb. (Show)
   Je n'ai plus de sensations dans une partie de la main ou du bras.
   (Montrer)
❏ I have pain. (Refer to Visual Pain Scale)
   J'ai mal. (Voir l'échelle de douleur)
❏ I have dislocated this shoulder before.
   Je me suis déjà luxé cette épaule.
❏ I have a prior injury to this same shoulder _____ months ago.
   Je me suis déjà fait mal à cette épaule il y a _____ mois.
❏ I have had surgery on this shoulder.
   J'ai déjà subi une opération de cette épaule.
❏ I last ate or drank _____ hours ago.
   J'ai mangé ou bu pour la dernière fois il y a _____ heures.
❏ I have taken acetaminophen (Tylenol).
   J'ai pris de l'acétaminophène (Tylenol).
❏ I have taken ibuprofen.
   J'ai pris de l'ibuprofène.
❏ I have taken another medicine: _____.
   J'ai pris un autre medicament: _____.
❏ I also have other injuries. (Show where they are)
   J'ai également mal à d'autres endroits du corps. (Préciser les
   zones concernées)

Elbow, Arm, or Wrist Injury

A fall onto an outstretched arm is a common cause of a broken wrist or elbow. The middle part of the forearm is more likely to be broken by a direct blow to the area. The elbow or wrist can start hurting without trauma due to inflammation of the tendons or bursa (lubricating sacs). This is very common with repeated movements, such as in tennis elbow.

Les blessures aux coude, bras, ou poignet

Une chute sur un bras tendu est une cause fréquente de fracture du poignet ou du coude. La partie centrale de l'avant-bras risque davantage de se casser sous l'effet d'un coup porté directement sur cette zone. Le coude ou le poignet peuvent commencer à être douloureux sans qu'il y ait eu traumatisme à cause d'une inflammation des tendons ou des bourses synoviales (liquide synovial). Cela est très fréquent dans le cas de mouvements répétés, comme pour les synovites du coude (tennis elbow).

Check only those questions to which you answer YES.
Cochez seulement les questions auxquelles vous répondez OUI.

Complaint
Symptômes

❏ I have injured my elbow. (Demonstrate)
  Je me suis fait mal au coude. (Démontrer)
❏ I have injured my forearm.
  Je me suis fait mal à l'avant-bras.
❏ I have injured my wrist.
  Je me suis fait mal au poignet.
❏ My arm hurts but I have not injured it.
  J'ai mal au bras mais je ne me suis pas blessé(e) au bras.
❏ I think it is:
  Je pense qu'il est:
    ❏ broken.
      cassé.
    ❏ sprained.
      foulé.

❏ bruised.
  contusionné.
❏ The problem started _____ minutes/hours/days ago.
  Le problème a débuté il y a _____ minutes/heures/jours.
❏ I fell down.
  Je suis tombé(e).
❏ I fell _____ feet. (1 foot = 0.30 meters)
  Je suis tombé(e) d'une hauteur de _____ centimètres/mètres.
❏ My arm was against my side when I fell. (Show)
  J'avais le bras le long du corps quand je suis tombé(e). (Montrer)
❏ My arm was above my head when I fell.
  J'avais le bras levé au-dessus de la tête quand je suis tombé(e).
❏ I can move my wrist/elbow.
  Je peux bouger le poignet/coude.
❏ I cannot move my wrist/elbow.
  Je ne peux pas bouger le poignet/coude.
❏ My hand feels normal.
  J'ai des sensations normales dans la main.
❏ Part of my hand feels asleep (numb). (Show)
  Je n'ai plus de sensations dans une partie de la main. (Montrer)
❏ I also have a cut on this arm. (Show)
  Je me suis également coupé(e) à ce bras (Montrer)
❏ I have pain. (Refer to Visual Pain Scale)
  J'ai mal. (Voir l'échelle de douleur)
❏ I injured this same extremity _____ months ago.
  Je me suis déjà fait mal à cette extrémité il y a _____ mois.
❏ I have had surgery on this extremity.
  J'ai déjà subi une opération de cette extrémité.
❏ I last ate or drank _____ hours ago.
  J'ai mangé ou bu pour la dernière fois il y a _____ heures.
❏ I have taken acetaminophen (Tylenol).
  J'ai pris de l'acétaminophène (Tylenol).
❏ I have taken ibuprofen.
  J'ai pris de l'ibuprofène.
❏ I have taken another medicine: _____.

J'ai pris un autre medicament: _____.

❏ I also have other injuries. (Show where the injuries are.)
J'ai également mal à d'autres endroits. (Préciser les zones concernées.)

Hand Injury

The hand is very complex. Seemingly minor injuries can be serious. Its 23 bones may be broken or dislocated. Lacerations can injure tendons or nerves. A tendon can rupture without a laceration, leaving a finger without function.

Les blessures à la main

La main est très complexe. Des blessures en apparence mineures peuvent, en fait, être graves. Les 23 os de la main peuvent se fracturer ou se luxer. Les coupures peuvent provoquer des lésions aux tendons et aux nerfs. Il peut y avoir rupture d'un tendon sans déchirure, entraînant la perte de motricité du doigt.

Check only those questions to which you answer YES.
Cochez seulement les questions auxquelles vous répondez OUI.

Complaint
Symptômes
❏ I have injured my hand.
Je me suis fait mal à la main.
❏ I have injured my right-hand finger(s)/thumb.
Je me suis fait mal au(x) doigt(s) de la main droite pouce.
❏ I have injured my left-hand finger(s)/thumb.
Je me suis fait mal au(x) doigt(s) de la main gauche pouce.
❏ My hand/finger hurts but I have not injured it.
J'ai mal à la main/au doigt mais je ne me suis pas blessé(e) à cet endroit-là.
❏ I think it is:
Je pense qu'elle/il est:
   ❏ broken.
   cassé(e).
   ❏ sprained.

foulé(e).

❏ bruised.

contusionné(e).

❏ I have a cut on this hand/finger.

Je me suis coupé à cette main/à ce doigt.

❏ It happened _____ minutes/hours/days ago.

Le problème a débuté il y a _____ minutes/heures/jours.

❏ I fell down.

Je suis tombé(e).

❏ I fell _____ feet. (1 foot = 0.30 meters)

Je suis tombé(e) d'une hauteur de _____ centimètres/mètres.

❏ My hand feels normal.

J'ai des sensations normales dans la main.

❏ Part of my hand feels like it's asleep (numb). (Demonstrate)

Je n'ai plus de sensations dans une partie de la main.

(Démontrer)

❏ I cannot move my finger(s).

Je ne peux plus bouger le(s) doigts(s).

❏ I have pain. (Refer to Visual Pain Scale)

J'ai mal. (Voir l'échelle de douleur)

❏ I injured this same extremity _____ months ago.

Je me suis déjà blessé à cette extrémité il y a _____ mois.

❏ I have had surgery on this extremity.

J'ai déjà subi une opération de cette extrémité.

❏ I last ate or drank _____ hours ago.

J'ai mangé ou bu pour la dernière fois il y a _____ heures.

❏ I have taken acetaminophen (Tylenol).

J'ai pris de l'acétaminophène (Tylenol).

❏ I have taken ibuprofen.

J'ai pris de l'ibuprofène.

❏ I have taken another medicine: _____.

J'ai pris d'autres medicaments: _____.

❏ I also have other injuries. (Show where the injuries are.)

J'ai mal à d'autres endroits du corps. (Préciser les zones

concernées.)

Environmental Injuries: Frostbite and Cold Injuries

Frostbite is the freezing of skin and deeper tissue caused by exposure to cold. It is most common on the face, ears, fingers, and toes. Frostnip is a less severe cold injury in which the tissue has not actually frozen. Frostbite appears initially as pale skin. It can progress to blistered or even blackened skin. Exposure to wet conditions makes this worse.

Treatment involves rapid warming, preferably with warm water, and pain medication. Warming should not be done at all until no risk of refreezing is present. The skin may look very bad after warming but no removal of what may appear to be dead skin (except blisters) should be done for several weeks. The injury is often not as extensive as it looks.

Hypothermia is a body temperature of less than 35° C (95° F). Treatment involves removing the person's wet clothing and rewarming him/her.

Les blessures liées au milieu: gelures et blessures dues au froid

Les gelures profondes correspondent à une congélation de la peau et des tissus sous-cutanés si l'on reste trop longtemps au froid. Elles se produisent le plus souvent sur le visage, les oreilles, les doigts et les orteils. Les gelures superficielles sont des blessures dues au froid moins graves qui n'entraînent pas la congélation des tissus sous-cutanés. Les gelures profondes se manifestent tout d'abord par une peau pâle. Elles peuvent ensuite évoluer et provoquer des ampoules sur la peau et même un noircissement de la peau. Ces caractéristiques s'accentuent par temps humide.

Le traitement des gelures consiste à réchauffer rapidement la peau, de préférence avec de l'eau chaude et des médicaments contre la douleur. Il ne faut absolument pas réchauffer la peau s'il subsiste un risque quelconque de re-congélation. Il se peut que la peau soit très vilaine après avoir été réchauffée mais il ne faut en aucun cas enlever les peaux qui semblent mortes (à l'exception des ampoules) pendant plusieurs semaines. La blessure n'est souvent pas aussi importante qu'elle ne le paraît.

L'hypothermie est une température du corps qui se situe au-dessous de 35° C (95° F). Le traitement de l'hypothermie nécessite d'enlever tous les vêtements mouillés et de réchauffer le corps.

Check only those questions to which you answer YES.
Cochez seulement les questions auxquelles vous répondez OUI.

Complaint
Symptômes
❏ I think I have frostbite.
  Je pense que j'ai une gelure.
❏ I think I have hypothermia.
  Je pense que je fais de l'hypothermie.
❏ I have been exposed to the cold for _____ minutes/hours/days.
  Je suis reste(e) au froid pendant pour _____ minutes/heures/jours.
❏ The injury involves my:
  La blessure se situe au niveau:
  ❏ ears.
    des oreilles.
  ❏ face.
    du visage.
  ❏ fingers (of right/left hand).
    des doigts (main droite/main gauche).
  ❏ toes (of right/left foot).
    des orteils (pied droit/pied gauche).
  ❏ feet (right/left).
    des pieds (droit/gauche).
❏ I have pain. (Refer to Visual Pain Scale)
  J'ai mal. (Voir l'échelle de douleur)
❏ I also have other injuries. (Show where the injuries are)
  J'ai également mal à d'autres endroits. (Indiquer les zones
  concernées)
❏ I have tried to warm the skin.
  J'ai essayé de réchauffer la peau.
❏ I have not tried to warm the skin.
  Je n'ai pas essayé de réchauffer la peau.
❏ I have taken acetaminophen (Tylenol).
  J'ai pris de l'acétaminophène (Tylenol).
❏ I have taken ibuprofen.
  J'ai pris de l'ibuprofène.

❏ I have taken another medicine(s): _____.
   J'ai pris d'autres medicaments: _____.
❏ I have had previous frostbite to the same area.
   J'ai déjà eu des gelures au même endroit.
❏ I have had frostbite to a different area.
   J'ai déjà eu des gelures à un endroit différent.

Heat Exhaustion and Heat Stroke (Hyperthermia)
Heat exhaustion and heat stroke are common events in travelers. They are more likely to occur in individuals with poor physical conditioning or who have not had appropriate acclimatization to heat. Limited access to fluids and salt also result in heat-related illnesses.

Les coups de chaleur (hyperthermie)
Les coups de chaleur sont des phénomènes courants chez les gens qui voyagent beaucoup. Ils surviennent généralement chez des individus en mauvaise forme physique ou ne s'étant pas acclimatés convenablement à la chaleur. Des difficultés pour se procurer des fluides et du sel provoquent aussi des maladies liées à la chaleur.

Check only those questions to which you answer YES.
Cochez seulement les questions auxquelles vous répondez OUI.

Complaint
Symptômes
❏ I think I have "heat stroke."
   Je pense que j'ai eu un "coup de chaleur."
❏ I have fatigue and lethargy.
   Je me send fatigué(e) et léthargique.
❏ I feel weak.
   Je me sens faible.
❏ I have dizziness.
   J'ai de vertiges.
❏ I have had had nausea.
   J'ai eu des nausées.
❏ I have had vomiting.
   J'ai vomi.

❏ I have aches in my muscles.
  J'ai des courbatures dans les muscles.
❏ I have a headache.
  J'ai mal à la tête.
❏ I have profuse sweating.
  Je transpire abondamment.
❏ I have not been sweating.
  Je ne transpire pas.
❏ I can feel my heart race.
  Je sens mon cœur battre à toute vitesse.
❏ I feel like I am passing out.
  J'ai l'impression que je vais m'évanouir.
❏ I have passed out.
  Je me suis évanoui(e).
❏ I do not feel as if I can walk normally.
  J'ai l'impression de ne pas marcher normalement.
❏ I have been confused.
  J'ai l'esprit confus.
❏ I am very thirsty.
  J'ai très soif.
❏ I have numbness and tingling in my right/left arms/legs.
  J'ai une sensation d'engourdissement et de picotement dans
    le/la/les bras/jambes(s). droit(e)/gauche.
❏ I have had a recent fever. (Refer to Temperature Scale)
  J'ai eu récemment de la fièvre. (Voir l'échelle de température)
❏ My fever was _____ minutes/hours/days ago.
  J'ai eu de la fièvre il y a _____ minutes/heures/jours.
❏ I have been using alcohol regularly.
  Je consomme de l'alcool régulièrement.
❏ I have been staying in a facility that does not have air conditioning.
  Je loge dans un endroit qui n'est pas climatisé.
❏ I have had limited access to water and fluids.
  J'ai eu des difficultés à me procurer de l'eau et des fluides.
❏ The above problem has been present for _____ minutes/hours/days.
  J'ai le problème ci-dessus depuis _____ minutes/heures/jours.

❑ My urine output has decreased.
  Mon débit urinaire a diminué.

Rash

Dermatologic diseases are based upon careful visual inspection by a physician. The following information will allow you to provide the healthcare professional with information regarding its history. Please be as accurate as possible. Previous treatments with other medications that have been successful and those which have been unsuccessful are important historical data.

Rashes are an extremely common problem, accounting for approximately seven percent of all outpatient visits to physicians. Medical history as well as medications (new and old) are of importance in relating medical history to medical professionals.

It is important to inform the physician as to the distribution of the rash, the history regarding its onset and original locations and whether it itches. Your recent travel (within the past seven days) and any exposure to chemicals are also important.

Les eruptions cutanees

Les maladies dermatologiques sont déterminées par un examen visuel attentif pratiqué par le médecin. Les informations suivantes vous permettront de fournir à votre professionnel de la santé des renseignements concernant le développement de cette maladie. Veuillez être aussi précis que possible. Les traitements antérieurs avec d'autres médicaments qui ont réussi, ainsi que ceux qui n'ont pas réussi, sont des renseignements importants sur vos antécédents dermatologiques.

Les éruptions cutanées sont un problème extrêmement courant qui représente environ 7% de l'ensemble des visites médicales effectuées par des patients en consultation externe. Les antécédents médicaux ainsi que les médicaments (nouveaux et anciens) sont très importants dans la transmission des renseignements médicaux aux professionnels de la santé.

Il est important d'informer le médecin de la répartition de l'éruption cutanée, de préciser la façon dont elle a débuté et les endroits du corps où elle s'est manifestée en premier, et de mentionner si elle provoque des démangeaisons. Vos déplacements récents (dans les sept derniers jours) ainsi que tout contact avec des produits chimiques sont également importants.

Check only those questions to which you answer YES.
Cochez seulement les questions auxquelles vous répondez OUI.

Complaint
Symptômes
❏ I have a rash.
  J'ai une éruption cutanée.
❏ The rash has been present for _____ hours/days.
  J'ai cette éruption cutanée depuis _____ heures/jours.
❏ The lesion contained fluid.
  La lésion contenait un fluide.
❏ The lesion broke open. This happened _____ minutes/hours/days
  ago.
  La lésion s'est ouverte. Cela s'est produit il y a _____
  minutes/heures/jours.
❏ The lesion's fluid was clear.
  Le fluide de la lésion était clair.
❏ The lesion's fluid looked infected.
  Le fluide de la lésion semblait infecté.
❏ The lesion's fluid contained blood.
  Le fluide de la lésion contenait du sang.
❏ I have used the following treatments: (show the physician which
  treatments).
  J'ai utilisé les traitements suivants: (montrer au médecin ces
  traitements).
❏ The lesion was treated successfully.
  La lésion a été traitée avec succès.
❏ The lesion was not treated successfully.
  La lésion n'a pas été traitée avec succès.
❏ I have used the following cream: (show the medication/cream).
  J'ai utilisé cette crème-ci: (montrer le médicament/la crème).
❏ The lesion is itchy.
  La lésion me démange.
❏ The lesion is painful.
  La lésion est douloureuse.
❏ The lesion bleeds.
  La lésion saigne.

❏ I have a family history of similar problems. My mother/father/
   sister/brother/cousins have similar problems.
   Il y a des problèmes analogues dans ma famille. Mon/ma/mes
   mere/père/sœur/frère/cousins ont des problèmes analogues.
❏ I have been exposed to someone with the same rash.
   J'ai été en contact avec quelqu'un qui avait la même éruption
   cutanée.
❏ I have had this rash before.
   J'ai déjà eu une éruption cutanée comme celle-ci.
❏ It was treated with: (show name of medication).
   On m'a traité(e) à/au: (indiquer au médecin le nom du
   médicament).
❏ I have traveled to the following areas recently:
   Je me suis rendu(e) aux endroits suivants récemment:

Date: _____   Location: _____

Date: _____   Lieu: _____

Date: _____   Location:_____

Date: _____   Lieu: _____

Date: _____   Location: _____

Date: _____   Lieu:_____

Date: _____   Location:_____

Date: _____   Lieu: _____

Date: _____   Location: _____

Date: _____   Lieu: _____

Lacerations

Every laceration is unique and it is difficult to describe which need to
be repaired with sutures, glue, or special bandages. Every laceration
does need to be properly cleaned. It is generally the width and length

of the cut rather than the depth that determines the need for stitches. Every laceration will heal without stitches, even very large ones. It may take an extremely long time to heal and there is a risk of infection with open wounds. There may be associated serious injuries such as nerve, joint, or tendon injuries that need attention as well. If a laceration is going to be fixed it should be done within approximately 16 hours. This is a guideline and may be altered in special circumstances. A laceration should be cleansed with soap and clean water. Peroxide, iodine, or alcohol should not be used. A general "rule of thumb" is that if you are asking yourself if you need stitches you should have it checked.

Les coupures
Toutes les coupures sont différentes, et c'est pourquoi il est difficile de décrire quel type de coupure nécessite d'être traité par des points de suture, une colle biologique ou un pansement particulier. Toute coupure doit être nettoyée avec soin. C'est généralement la largeur et la longueur de la coupure, et non sa profondeur, qui déterminent la nécessité d'avoir recours à des points de suture. Toute coupure peut guérir sans point de suture, même les très grosses coupures. Néanmoins, cela peut mettre énormément de temps à guérir et les blessures ouvertes entraînent toujours des risques d'infection. Ces coupures peuvent s'accompagner de lésions graves aux nerfs, aux articulations ou aux tendons qui nécessitent d'être examinées également. Si une coupure doit être soignée, il faut que cela soit fait dans les 16 heures qui suivent, approximativement. C'est ce que l'on recommande, mais il peut en être différemment dans des cas exceptionnels. Il faut nettoyer une coupure avec du savon et de l'eau bien propre, et ne pas utiliser de peroxyde, d'iode ou d'alcool. En règle générale, si vous vous demandez s'il y a besoin ou non de points de suture, faites examiner votre coupure.

Check only those questions to which you answer YES.
Cochez seulement les questions auxquelles vous répondez OUI.

Complaint
Symptômes
❏ I have a laceration (cut).
 Je me suis coupé(e).

❏ I have more than one laceration. I have _____ (give number). (Show)

Je me suis coupé(e) à plusieurs endroits. J'ai _____ (indiquer le nombre). (Montrer)

❏ The problem started _____ minutes/hours/days ago.

Le problème a débuté il y a _____ minutes/heures/jours.

❏ I was cut with:

Je me suis coupé(e) avec:

  ❏ glass.

    du verre.

  ❏ a knife.

    un couteau.

  ❏ a stick.

    un baton.

  ❏ in a fall.

    en tombant.

  ❏ other: _____

    autres: _____

❏ The object was clean.

L'objet était proper.

❏ The object was dirty.

L'objet était sale.

❏ I had a tetanus immunization _____ years ago.

Je me suis fait vacciner contre le tétanos il y a _____ ans.

❏ I have pain. (Refer to Visual Pain Scale)

J'ai mal. (Voir l'échelle de douleur)

❏ I cannot move part of my body. (Demonstrate)

Je ne peux pas bouger certaines parties du corps. (Démontrer)

❏ I cannot feel part of my body. (Demonstrate)

Je n'ai plus de sensations dans certaines parties du corps. (Démontrer)

❏ The cut bled a lot.

La coupure saignait abondamment.

❏ The cut did not bleed much.

La coupure ne saignait pas beaucoup.

Electrical Injuries

Electrical injuries are nearly always accidental. Though generally preventable, these events can occur unexpectedly. Included in this section are lightning-induced injuries.

The mechanism associated with electrical injuries involves the direct effect of electrical current on body tissues. The conversion of electrical energy to thermal injury may result in deep or superficial burns. Blunt injuries occur after a lightning strike. These injuries are usually due to a fall and electrically-induced muscle contractions.

Whenever possible, it is important to know the source of the electrical shock, the presence of either alternating current (AC) or direct current (DC), and any assciated events such as loss of consciousness or seizures. Please note that in Europe, most home voltage is 220.

Les électrocutions

Les électrocutions sont presque toujours accidentelles. Bien qu'on puisse généralement les éviter, ces accidents peuvent survenir sans que l'on s'y attende. Cette section comporte aussi les blessures dues à la foudre.

Le mécanisme des blessures associées aux électrocutions implique l'effet direct du courant électrique sur les tissus corporels. La conversion de l'énergie électrique en blessure thermique peut entraîner des brûlures profondes et superficielles. Des blessures brutales surviennent lorsque la foudre tombe. Elles sont généralement dues à une chute ou à des contractions musculaires causées par la décharge électrique.

Dans la mesure du possible, il est important de connaître la source de la décharge électrique, la présence soit de courant alternatif (CA), soit de courant continu (CD), et tous les autres phénomènes associés tels que perte de connaissance ou attaques cérébrales. Veuillez noter qu'en Europe, la plupart des voltages domestiques sont de 220 volts.

Check only those questions to which you answer YES.
Cochez seulement les questions auxquelles vous répondez OUI.

Complaint
Symptômes
❑ I have had an electrical injury.

Je me suis électrocuté(e).

❑ This injury occurred _____ minutes/hours ago.
  La blessure est survenue il y a _____ minutes/heures.

❑ I was shocked by standard house current.
  J'ai reçu une décharge électrique provenant du courant domestique.

❑ The voltage was less than 1000 volts.
  Le voltage était inférieur à 1000 volts.

❑ The voltage was greater than 1000 volts.
  Le voltage était supérieur à 1000 volts.

❑ The shock occurred here. (Indicate area of initial electrical injury)
  La décharge s'est produite ici. (Indiquer l'endroit de l'électrocution initiale)

❑ A flash (arc) burn occurred.
  Il y a eu une brûlure (arc) subite.

❑ I saw flames.
  J'ai vu des flammes.

❑ I was struck by lightning.
  J'ai été frappé(e) par la foudre.

❑ I was wet when the injury occurred.
  J'étais mouillé(e) au moment de la blessure.

❑ I am burned. (Indicate location of burn injury)
  J'ai une brûlure. (Indiquer l'endroit de la brûlure)

❑ I passed out.
  Je me suis évanoui(e).

❑ I passed out for _____ minutes/hours.
  Je me suis évanoui(e) pendant _____ minutes/heures.

❑ I had a seizure.
  J'ai eu une attaque cérébrale.

❑ I have a pacemaker.
  J'ai un pacemaker.

❑ I have chest pain. (Fill out the Chest Pain Section if you feel it is necessary.)
  J'ai une douleur à la poitrine. (Complétez la section concernant les douleurs à la poitrine si vous le jugez nécessaire)

❑ I have prosthetic joints. (Indicate which joints)
  J'ai des prothèses articulaires. (Indiquer quelles articulations)

❏ I have heart disease.

J'ai une maladie cardiaque.

❏ I have aches in my muscles and joints. (Indicate muscles and joint area)

J'ai des douleurs musculaire et articulaires. (Indiquer la zone musculaire et articulaire)

❏ I have been passing red urine.

J'urine du sang.

❏ I have weakness.

Je me sens faible.

❏ I cannot recall what happened.

Je ne me souviens plus de ce qui s'est passé.

❏ I cannot see.

Je ne vois plus rien.

❏ I have ringing in my ears.

J'ai une sonnerie dans les oreilles.

❏ I have dizziness.

J'ai des vertiges.

❏ I have abdominal pain.

J'ai des douleurs abdominales.

❏ I have a history of weak bones (osteoporosis).

J'ai déjà eu des insuffisances osseuses (ostéoporose).

❏ I have a history of ulcers.

J'ai déjà eu des ulcères.

❏ I have skeletal pain. (Indicate location)

J'ai des douleurs dans les os. (Indiquer à quel endroit)

Prescription Medications

Prescription medications vary from country to country. The list below is derived from the top sales figures worldwide for prescription medications. Various preparations are sold in each country based upon regulatory statutes. All the variations of medications cannot be accommodated in a text of this size.

The list is organized according to the major indication (allergy, analgesics, etc.) of the drugs. Following each drug is the generic name and brand name. Within the parentheses, are the translations for the medication, if available. The dosages are for United States FDA approved indications. The dose may vary in foreign countries. The indication for the drug is provided to help you verify that you have selected the correct drug. Many medications are available in the United Staes but not in foreign states and vice versa. The drug prescribed in the United States will likely have an equivalent, but different, name.

Remember, it is always important to complete the Medication and Allergy Section in the front of the book. Prior to departure, you should have a complete list of medications and allergies, preferably on your physician's stationary, placed in a separate location.

Allergy Medications
(Allergie Medicaments)

Allegra
    Generic/Dose: fexofenadine (féxofenadine chlorhydrate) 30 mg,
                   60 mg, 180 mg
    Indication: allergy (allergie)

Allegra D
    Generic/Dose: fexofenadine HCL (féxofenadine) 60mg
                   pseudoephedrine HCL (pseudoéphédrine sulfate)
                   120 mg
    Indication: allergy (allergie)

Claritin
    Generic/Dose: loratidine (loratidine) 10 mg
    Indication: allergy (allergie)

Claritin D
    Generic/Dose: loratidine (loratidine) 5 mg pseudoephedrine
                  (pseudephedrine) 120 mg
    Indication: allergy (allergie)

Flonase
    Generic/Dose: fluticasone propionate (fluticasone) 50 mcg/spray
    Indication: allergy (allergie)

Nasonex
    Generic/Dose: mometasone furoate (mométasone furoate
                  monohydrate) 50 mcg/spray
    Indication: allergy (allergie)

Zyrtec
    Generic/Dose: certrizine (cértirizine) 5 mg, 10 mg
    Indication: allergy (allergie)

Analgesics
(Analgésique)

NB: NSAID means Nonsteroidal Anti-inflammatory Drug

Celebrex
    Generic/Dose: celecoxib (célécoxib) 100 mg, 200 mg
    Indication: analgesic
                  NSAID

Ultram
    Generic/Dose: tramadol (tramadol chlohydrate) 50 mg
    Indication: analgesic (analgésique)

Motrin
    Generic/Dose: ibuprofen (ibuprofène) 400 mg
    Indication: analgesic (analgésique)
                  NSAID

Neurontin
    Generic/Dose: gabapentin (gabapentine) 100mg, 300 mg, 400
                  mg, 600 mg

Indication: analgesic (analgésique)
                seizure (attaque brusque)

Relafen
  Generic/Dose: nabumetone (nabumétone) 500 mg, 750 mg
  Indication: analgesic (analgésique)
                NSAID
Naprosyn
  Generic/Dose: naproxen (naproxène sel de Na) 375 mg, 500 mg
  Indication: analgesic (analgésique)
                NSAID

Vioxx
  Generic/Dose: rofecoxib (rofécoxib) 12.5 mg, 25 mg
  Indication: analgesic (analgésique)
                NSAID

Roxicet
  Generic/Dose: oxycodone (oxycodone chlorhydrate) 5 mg
                acetominophen (paracétamol) 500 mg
  Indication: analgesic (analgésique)
                narcotic (narcotique)

Valium
  Generic/Dose: diazepam (diazepam) 2 mg, 5 mg, 10 mg
  Indication: anxiety (anxiété)

OxyContin
  Generic/Dose: oxycodone (oxycodone chlorhydrate) 10mg, 20mg,
                40mg, 80mg
  Indication: analgesic (analgésique)
                narcotic (narcotique)

Arthrotec (multiple preparations)
  Generic/Dose: diclenofac (diclofénac sel de Na) 50 mg/
                misoprostol (misoprostol) 200 mcg
                diclenofac (diclofénac sel de Na) 75 mg/
                misoprostol (misoprostol) 200 mcg
  Indication: osteoarthritis (ostéoathrite)
                NSAID
                prostaglandin

Vicodin
    Generic/Dose: hydrocodone bitartrate 5 mg acetaminophen
                500 mg
    Indication: analgesic (analgésique)
                narcotic (narcotique)

Demerol
    Generic/Dose: meperidine (mépéridine = péthidine) 50 mg,
                100 mg
    Indication: analgesic (analgésique)
                narcotic (narcotique)

Antibiotics
(Antibiotique)

Amoxicillin
    Generic/Dose: amoxicillin (amoxcilline trihydrate/acide
                clavulanique sel de K) 250 mg, 500 mg
    Indication: antibiotic (antibiotique)

Zithromax – Z pack
    Generic/Dose: azithromycin (azithromycine dihydrate) 250 mg,
                600 mg
    Indication: antibiotic (antibiotique)

Augmentin (multiple preparations)
    Generic/Dose: amoxicillin (amoxcilline trihydrate) 250 mg
                clavulinic acid(acide clavulanique sel de K)
                125 mg
                amoxicillin (amoxcilline trihydrate) 500 mg
                clavulinic acid (acide clavulanique sel de K)
                125 mg
                amoxicillin (amoxcilline trihydrate) 875 mg
                clavulinic acid (acide clavulanique sel de K) 125
    Indication: antibiotic (antibiotique)

Cipro
    Generic/Dose: ciprofloxacin (ciprofloxacine chlorhydrate
                monohydrate) 100 mg, 250 mg, 500 mg, 750 mg
    Indication: antibiotic (antibiotique)

Keflex
 Generic/Dose: Cephalexin (céfalexine monohydrate) 250 mg, 500 mg
 Indication: antibiotic (antibiotique)

Bactrim
 Generic/Dose: trimethoprim (triméthoprime) 160 mg
  sulfamethoxazole (sulfaméthoxazole) 800 mg
 Indication: antibiotic (antibiotique)

Biaxin
 Generic/Dose: clarithromycin (clarithromycine) 250 mg, 500 mg
 Indication: antibiotic (antibiotique)

Diflucan
 Generic/Dose: fluconazole (fluconazole) 50 mg, 100 mg, 200 mg
 Indication: antifungal

Levaquin
 Generic/Dose: levofloxacin (lévofoxacine hemihydrate) 250 mg,
  500 mg
 Indication: antibiotic (antibiotique)

Cefzil
 Generic/Dose: cefprozil (cefprozil) 250 mg, 500 mg
 Indication: antibiotic (antibiotique)

Bactroban
 Generic/Dose: mupirocin (mupirocine sel de Ca) 2% cream/
  ointment
 Indication: antibiotic (antibiotique)

Macrobid
 Generic/Dose: nitrofurantoin monohydrate (nitrofurantoïne) 75 mg
  macrocrystals 25 mg
 Indication: antibiotic (antibiotique)

Ery-Tab
 Generic/Dose: erythromycin (érythromycine éthylsuccinate) 250 mg
 Indication: antibiotic (antibiotique)
  extended release

Cardiology Medications

Diovan
  Generic/Dose: valsartan (valsartan) 80 mg, 160 mg
  Indication: hypertension (hypertension)

Avapro
  Generic/Dose: irbersartan (irbesartan) 75 mg, 150 mg, 300 mg
  Indication: hypertension (hypertension)

Cozaar
  Generic/Dose: losartan (losartan sel de K) 25mg, 50 mg, 100 mg
  Indication: hypertension (hypertension)

Lipitor
  Generic/Dose: atorvastin (atorvastatine sel de Ca trihydrate)
                10 mg, 20 mg, 40 mg
  Indication: hyperlipidemia (hyperlipémie)
                hypercholesterolemia (hypercholesterolémie)

Norvasc
  Generic/Dose: amiodipine besylate (amlodipine bésilate) 2.5 mg,
                5 mg, 10 mg
  Indication: hypertension (hypertension)
                angina (angine)

Lanoxin
  Generic/Dose: digoxin (digoxine) 0.125 mg, 0.25 mg
  Indication: arrhythmias

Zestril
  Generic/Dose: lisinopril (lisinopril dihydrate) 2.5 mg, 5 mg,
                10 mg, 20 mg, 30 mg, 40 mg
  Indication: hypertension (hypertension)

Zocor
  Generic/Dose: simvastin (simvastatine) 5 mg, 10 mg, 20 mg,
                40 mg 80 mg
  Indication: hypercholesterolemia

Coumadin
  Generic/Dose: warfarin (warfarine sel de Na) 1 mg, 2 mg, 2.5
                 mg, 3.0 mg, 4.0 mg, 5.0 mg, 6.0 mg, 7.5 mg, 10 mg
  Indication: anticoagulation

Vasotec
  Generic/Dose: enalapril maleate (énalapril maleate) 2.5mg, 5 mg,
                 10 mg, 20.0 mg
  Indication: hypertension (hypertension)

Lasix
  Generic/Dose: furosemide (furosémide) 20 mg, 40 mg, 80 mg
  Indication: hypertension (hypertension)
                 diuretic (diurétique)

Pravachol
  Generic/Dose: pravastatin (pravastatine sel de Na) 10 mg, 20 mg,
                 40 mg
  Indication: hypercholesterolemia (hypercholestérolemie)

K-Dur
  Generic/Dose: potassium chloride (potassium chlorue) 10, 20 mg
  Indication: potassium replacement

Tenoromin
  Generic/Dose: atenolol (aténolol) 25 mg, 50 mg, 100 mg
  Indication: hypertension (hypertension)
                 angina (angine)

Accupril
  Generic/Dose: quinapril (quinapril chlorhydrate) 5 mg, 10 mg,
                 20 mg, 40 mg
  Indication: hypertension (hypertension)

Cardiazem CD
  Generic/Dose: diltiazem (diltiazem chlorhydrate) 120 mg,
                 180 mg, 240 mg, 300 mg
  Indication: hypertension (hypertension)

Toprol
  Generic/Dose: metoprolol (métoprolol succinate) 25 mg, 50 mg,

100 mg
Indication: hypertension (hypertension)

Dyazide
Generic/Dose: triamterene (triamtérène) 25 mg
     hydrochlorothiazide (hydrochlorothiazide) 37.5 mg
Indication: hypertension (hypertension)
     diuretic (diurétique)

Cardura
Generic/Dose: doxazosin (doxazosine mésilate) 1, 2, 4, 8 mg
Indication: hypertension (hypertension)

Lotensin
Generic/Dose: benazepril (bénazépril chlorhydrate) 5, 10, 20,
     40 mg
Indication: hypertension (hypertension)

Procardia XL
Generic/Dose: nifedipine (nifédipine) 10 mg, 20 mg
Indication: angina (angine)

HydroDiuril
Generic/Dose: hydrochlorothiazide (hydrochlorothiazide) 25 mg,
     50 mg, 100 mg
Indication: hypertension (hypertension)
     diuretic (diurétique)

Adalat CC
Generic/Dose: nifedipine (nifédipine) 10 mg, 20 mg
Indication: angina (angine)

Monopril
Generic/Dose: fosinopril (fosinopril sel de Na) 10 mg, 20 mg,
     40 mg
Indication: hypertension (hypertension)

Calan SR
Generic/Dose: verapamil (vérapamil chlorhydrate) 120 mg, 180
     mg, 240 mg

Indication: hypertension (hypertension)
extended release

Ziac (multiple preparations)
Generic/Dose: bisoprolol fumarate (bisoprolol hémifomarate) 2.5 mg
hydrochlorothiazide (hydrochlorothiazide) 6.25 mg
bisoprolol fumarate (bisoprolol hémifomarate)
5.0 mg
hydrochlorothiazide (hydrochlorothiazide) 6.25 mg
bisoprolol fumarate (bisoprolol hémifomarate)
s10 mg
hydrochlorothiazide (hydrochlorothiazide) 6.25 mg
Indication: hypertension (hypertension)
diuretic (diurétique)

Lescol
Generic/Dose: fluvastastin (fluvastatine sel de Na) 20 mg, 40 mg
Indication: hypercholesterolemia (hypercholesterolémie)

Plavix
Generic/Dose: clopidrogel bisulfate (clopidrogel) 75 mg
Indication: anticoagulant (anticoagulant)

Hyzaar (multiple preparations)
Generic/Dose: losartan (losartan sel de K) 50 mg
hydrochlorothiazide (hydrochlorthiazide) 12.5 mg
losartan (losartan sel de K) 100 mg
hydrochlorothiazide (hydrochlorothiazide) 25 mg
Indication: hypertension (hypertension)

Zestoretic (multiple preparations)
Generic/Dose: lisinopril (lisinopril dihydrate) 10 mg
hydrochlorothiazide (hydrochlorthiazide) 12.5 mg
lisinopril (lisinopril dihydrate) 20 mg
hydrochlorothiazide (hydrochlorthiazide) 12.5 mg
lisinopril (lisinopril dihydrate) 20 mg
hydrochlorothiazide (hydrochlorthiazide) 25 mg
Indication: hypertension (hypertension)
diuretic (diurétique)

ImDur
  Generic/Dose: isosorbide mononitrate (isosorbide 5-mononitrate)
              30 mg, 60 mg, 120 mg
  Indication: angina (angine)

Catapres
  Generic/Dose: clonidine hydrochlorate (clonidine chlorhydrate)
              0.1, 0.2, 0.3 mg
  Indication: hypertension (hypertension)

Inderal (multiple preparations)
Inderal
  Generic/Dose: propranolol (propranolol chlorhydrate) 10 mg,
              20 mg, 40 mg, 80 mg
  Indication: hypertension (hypertension)

Inderal LA
  Generic/Dose: propranolol (propranolol chlorhydrate) 60 mg
              80 mg, 120 mg, 160 mg
  Indication: hypertension (hypertension)
              extended release

Inderide (combination with diuretic hydrochlorothiazide (HCTZ)
  Generic/Dose: propranolol (propranolol chlorhydrate) 40 mg
              hydrochlorothiazide (hydrocholorothiazide) 25 mg
              propranolol (propranolol chlorhydrate) 80 mg
              hydrochlorothiazide (hydrochlorthiazide) 25 mg
  Indication: hypertension (hypertension)
              diuretic (diurétique)

Inderide LA Long-acting beta blocker with diuretic (HCTZ)
  Generic/Dose: propranolol (propranolol chlorhydrate) 80 mg
              hydrochlorothiazide (hydrochlorthiazide) 50 mg
              propranolol (propranolol chlorhydrate) 120 mg
              hydrochlorothiazide (hydrochlorthiazide) 50 mg
              propranolol (propranolol chlorhydrate) 180 mg
              hydrochlorothiazide (hydrochlorthiazide) 50 mg
  Indication: hypertension (hypertension)
              extended release
              diuretic (diurétique)

Lotrel (multiple preparations)
Generic/Dose: amiodipine (amlodipidine bésilate) 2.5 mg
benazepril (bénazépril chlorhydrate)10 mg
amiodipine (amlodipidine bésilate) 5 mg
benazepril (bénazépril chlorhydrate)10 mg
amiodipine (amlodipidine bésilate) 5 mg
benazepril (bénazépril chlorhydrate) 20 mg
Indication: hypertension (hypertension)

Nitrostat
Generic/Dose: nitroglycerine (nitroglycérine) 0.3 mg, 0.4 mg,
0.6 mg sublingual preparation
Indication: angina (angine)

Plendil
Generic/Dose: felodipine (félodipine) 2.5 mg, 5 mg, 10 mg
Indication: hypertension (hypertension)
calcium channel blocker

Lopid
Generic/Dose: gemfibrozil (gemfibrozil) 600 mg
Indication: hypertriglyceridemia (hyperlipémie)

Mevacor
Generic/Dose: lovastatin10 mg, 20 mg, 40 mg
Indication: hypercholesterolemia (hypercholesterolémie)

Tiazac
Generic/Dose: diltiazem (diltiazem chlorhydrate) 20 mg, 180 mg,
240 mg, 300 mg, 360 mg, 420 mg
Indication: hypertension (hypertension)
extended release

Altace
Generic/Dose: ramipril (ramipril) 1.25 mg, 2.5 mg, 5 mg, 10 mg
Indication: hypertension (hypertension)

Dermatology Medications

Lamisil
Generic/Dose: terbinafine (terbinafine chlorhydrate) 250 mg
Indication: cutaneous fungal infections

Endocrinology Medications

Amaryl
Generic/Dose: glimepiride (glimépiride) 1 mg, 2 mg, 4 mg
Indication: diabetes (diabète)

Premarin
Generic/Dose: conjugated estrogens (estrogénes sulfoconjugues
équins) 0.625 mg
medroxyprogesterone acetate (médroxyprogestérone acetate) 5.0 mg
Indication: menopause (mènopause)

Synthroid
Generic/Dose: levothyroxine (lévothyroxine sodique) 25 mcg,
50 mcg, 75 mcg, 88 mcg, 100 mcg, 112 mcg,
125 mcg, 150 mcg, 175 mcg, 200 mcg 300 mcg
Indication: hypothyroidism (hypothyroïdie)

Glucophage
Generic/Dose: metformin (metformine chlorhydrate) 500 mg,
850 mg, 1 gram
Indication: diabetes (diabète)

PremPro
Generic/Dose: conjugated estrogens (estrog_nes sulfoconjugués
équi) 0.625 mg
medroxyprogesterone acetate (médroxyprogestérone
acetate) 2.5 mg
Indication: menopause (mènopause)

Levoxyl
Generic/Dose: levothyroxine sodium (lévothyroxine sodique)

            25 mcg, 50 mcg, 75 mcg, 88 mcg, 100 mcg, 112
            mcg, 125 mcg, 137 mcg, 150 mcg, 175 mcg,
            200 mcg, 300 mcg
Indication: hypothyroidism (hypothyroïdie)

Prednisone
  Generic/Dose: prednisone (prednisone) multiple doses available
  Indication: immune suppression/multiple indications for use

Ortho Tricyclen
  Generic/Dose: norgestimate (norgestimate) 0.180 mg
               ethinylestradiol (éthinylestradiol) 0.035 mg
  Indication: contraception (contraception)

Glucotrol XL
  Generic/Dose: glipizide (glipizide) 5 mg, 10 mg
  Indication: diabetes (diabète)

Fosamax
  Generic/Dose: alendronate 5 mg, 10 mg, 40 mg
  Indication: osteoporosis (ostéoporose)

Triphasil (21 and 28 day regimens)
  Generic/Dose: ethinylestradiol (éthinylestradiol)
               levonorgestrel (lévonorgestrel)
                dose dependent upon the regimen prescribed
  Indication: contraception (contraception)

Ortho Novum 1/35
  Generic/Dose: northindrone (noréthistérone) 1 mg ethinylestradiol
               (éthinylestradiol) 35 mg
  Indication: contraception (contraception)

Ortho-Novum 1/50
  Generic/Dose: northindrone (noréthistérone) 1 mg
               mestranol 50 mg
  Indication: contraception (contraception)

Diabeta
  Generic/Dose: glyburide (glibenclamide) 1.25 mg, 2.5 mg,

5.0 mg

Indication: diabetes (diabète)

Lo/Ovral
Generic/Dose: noregestrel (lévonorgestrel) 0.3 mg
ethinylestradiol (éthinylestradiol)0.03 mg
Indication: contraception (contraception)

Evista
Generic/Dose: raloxifene hydrochloride (raloxiféne chlorhydrate)
60 mg
Indication: osteoporosis (ostéoporose)

Miacalcinin
Generic/Dose: calcitonin salmon (calcitonine synthétique savron)
220 IU/ml
Indication: osteoporosis (ostéoporose)

Desogen
Generic/Dose: desogrestrel (désogestrel) 0.15 mg esthinyl
estradi ol (éthinylestradiol) 0.03 mg
Indication: contraception (contraception)

Alesse
Generic/Dose: levonorgesterel (lévonorgestrel) 0.10 mg
ethinylestradiol (éthinylestradiol) 0.02 mg
Indication: contraception (contraception)

Necon
Generic/Dose: norethindrene (noréthistérone acetate) 0.5 mg
ethinylestradiol (éthinylestradiol) 35 mcg
Indication: contraception (contraception)

Necon 1/35
Generic/Dose: norethindrene (noréthistérone acétate) 1.0 mg
ethinylestradiol (éthinylestradiol) 35 mcg
Indication: contraception (contraception)

Estrace
Generic/Dose: estradiol (estradiol hémihydrate) 0.5 mg, 1.0 mg,

                    2.0 mg
    Indication: menopause (mènopause)

Levothroid
    Generic/Dose: levothyroxine (lévothyroxine sodique)
                    25 mcg, 50 mcg, 75 mcg, 88 mcg, 100 mcg, 112
                    mcg, 125 mcg, 137 mcg, 150 mcg, 175 mcg, 200
                    mcg, 300 mcg
    Indication: hypothyroidism (hypothyroïdie)

Cycrin
    Generic/Dose: medroxyprogesterone acetate (médroxy
                    progestérone acétate) 2.5 mg, 5.0 mg, 10 mg
    Indication: contraception (contraception)

Climara (multiple preparations)
    Generic/Dose: estradiol transdermal (estradiol hémihydrate)
                    Doses per patch: 2.0 mg (0.25 mg/day), 3.8 mg
                    (0.05 mg/day), 5.7 mg (0.075 mg/day), 7.6 mg
                    (0.1 mg/day)
    Indication: menopause (mènopause)

Gastrointestinal Medications

Prilosec 20 mg
    Generic/Dose: omeprazole (oméprazole) 10 mg, 20 mg, 40 mg
    Indication: ulcer (ulcére peptique) gastroesophageal reflux
                    disease (oesphagite)

Nexium
    Generic/Dose: esoprazole 40 mg
    Indication: ulcer (ulcére peptique) gastroesophageal reflux
                    disease (oesphagite)

Protonix
    Generic/Dose: pantoprazole (pantoprazole) 40 mg
    Indication: ulcer (ulcére peptique) gastroesophageal reflux
                    disease (oesphagite)
Prevacid
    Generic/Dose: lansoprazole (lansoprazole) 30 mg

Indication: ulcer (ulcére peptique) gastroesophageal reflux
              disease (oesphagite)

Aciphex
Generic/Dose: rabeprazole (rabéprazole sel de Na) 20 mg
Indication: ulcer (ulcére peptique) gastroesophageal reflux
              disease (oesphagite)

Pepcid
Generic/Dose: famotidine (famotidine) 20 mg, 40 mg
Indication: ulcer (ulcére peptique) gastroesophageal reflux
              disease (oesphagite)

Tagamet
Generic/Dose: cimetidine (cimétidine) 300 mg
Indication: ulcer (ulcére peptique) gastroesophageal reflux
              disease (oesphagite)

Zantac
Generic/Dose: ranitidine (ranitidine chlorhydrate) 75 mg, 150 mg
ndication: ulcer (ulcére peptique) gastroesophageal reflux
              disease (oesphagite)

Axid
Generic/Dose: nizatidine (nizatidine) 150 mg, 300 mg
Indication: sulcer (ulcére peptique) gastroesophageal reflux
              disease (oesphagite)

Intron A
Generic/Dose: interferon alpha 2b (various doses) (interféron
              alpha – 2b recombinant)
Indication: Hepatitis C (other oncology indications exist)

Rebetrol
Generic/Dose: ribavarin (ribavirine) weight based dosing
Indication: antiviral (combination therapy with interferon for
              Hepatitis C)

Rebetron
Generic/Dose: interferon/ribavarin combination (interféron alpha

– 2b recombinant ribavarine) weight based
dosing

Indication: Hepatitis C (HCV)

Oncology Medications

Tamoxifen
Generic/Dose: tamoxifen citrate (tamoxiféne citrate) 10 mg, 20 mg
Indication: breast cancer

Procrit
Generic/Dose: erythropoietin (époétine alpha) 20,000 units/ml
subcutaneous injection
Indication: anemia (anémie)

Neupogen
Generic/Dose: filgrastime (filgrastime) 300 mcg/ml
subcutaneous injection
Indication: leukopenia (leucopénie)

Ophthamology Medications

Tobradex
Generic/Dose: tobramycin/dexamethasone (tobramycine
sulfate/dexaméthason) eye drops
Indication: eye infection

Alphagan
Generic/Dose: brimonidine tartrate (brimonidine tartrate) 0.2%
Indication: glaucoma (glaucome)

Xalatan
Generic/Dose: latanoprost (latanoprost) 125 micrograms/2.5 ml
Indication: glaucoma (glaucome)

Neurologic Medications

Depakote
Generic/Dose: divalproex sodium (acid valproique sel de Na) 125
mg, 250 mg, 500 mg

Indication: seizure (attaque brusque)migraine headache
                    (migraine)

Dilantin
Generic/Dose: phenytoin (phénytoine) 30 mg, 100 mg
Indication: seizure (attaque brusque)

Imitrex
Generic/Dose: sumatriptan (sumatriptan succinate) 25 mg, 50 mg
Indication: migraine headache (migraine)

Aricept
Generic/Dose: donepezil (donépézil chlorhydrate) 5 mg, 10 mg
Indication: Alzheimer's disease (Maladie d'Alzheimer)

Psychiatric Medications

Prozac
Generic/Dose: fluoxetine HCl (fluoxétine chlorhydrate) 10 mg, 20
                    mg, 40 mg
Indication: depression (depression)

Zoloft
Generic/Dose: sertraline (sertraline chlorhydrate) 25 mg, 50 mg,
                    100 mg
Indication: depression (depression)

Paxil
Generic/Dose :paroxetine (paroxétine chlorhydrate) 10 mg, 20 mg,
                    30 mg, 40 mg
Indication: depression (depression)
                    anxiety (anxiété)

Ambien
Generic/Dose: zolpidem (zolpidem tartrate) 5 mg, 10 mg
Indication: insomnia (insomnie)

Alprazolam
Generic/Dose: alprazolam (alprazolam) 0.25 mg, 0.5 mg, 1 mg
Indication: anxiety (anxiété)

Wellbutrin SR
Generic/Dose: bupropion (bupropion chlorhydrate) 100 mg, 150 mg

Indication: depression (depression)
                extended release

Neurontin
  Generic/Dose: gabapentin (gabapentine) 100 mg, 300 mg, 400 mg
  Indication: seizure (attaque brusque)
               analgesic (analgésique)

Ativan
  Generic/Dose: lorazepam (lorazépam) 0.5 mg, 1.0 mg, 2.0 mg
  Indication: anxiety (anxiété)

Risperdal
  Generic/Dose: risperidone (rispéridone) 0.25 mg, 0.5 mg, 1 mg,
                2 mg, 3 mg
  Indication: schizophrenia (schizophrénie)

Klonopin
  Generic/Dose: clonazepam (clonazépam) 0.5 mg, 1.0 mg, 2.0 mg
  Indication: seizure (attaque brusque)

Elavil
  Generic/Dose: amitryptilline (amitryptyline chlorhydrate) 10 mg,
                25 mg, 50 mg, 75 mg, 100 mg, 150 mg
  Indication: depression (depression)

Buspar
  Generic/Dose: buspirone (buspirone chlorhydrate) 5 mg, 10 mg,
                15 mg, 30 mg
  Indication: anxiety (anxiété)

Celexa
  Generic/Dose: citalopram (citalopram bromhydrate) 20 mg, 40 mg
  Indication: depression (depression)

Effexor XR
  Generic/Dose: venlafaxine HCL (venlafaxine chlorhydrate) 25 mg,
                37.5 mg, 50 mg, 75 mg, 100 mg
  Indication: depression (depression)
               anxiety (anxiété)

Serzone
    Generic/Dose: nefazodone 50 mg, 100 mg, 150 mg, 200 mg, 250 mg
    Indication: depression (depression)

Adderal
    Generic/Dose: dextroamphetamine salts 5 mg, 10 mg, 20 mg, 30 mg
    Indication: attention deficit disorder

Concerta
    Generic/Dose: methylphenidate (méthylphenidate chlorhydrate)
                18 mg, 36 mg
    Indication: attention deficit disorder

Ritalin
    Generic/Dose: methylphenidate (méthylphenidate chlorhydrate) 5
                mg, 10 mg, 20 mg
    Indication: attention deficit disorder

Ritalin SR
    Generic/Dose: methylphenidate (méthylphenidate chlorhydrate)
                20 mg
    Indication: attention deficit disorder
                extended release

Restoril
    Generic/Dose: Temazepam (témazépam) 7.5 mg, 15 mg, 30 mg
    Indication: insomnia (insomnie)

Zyprexa
    Generic/Dose: olanzapine (olanzapine) 2.5 mg, 0.5 mg, 7.5 mg,
                10 mg
    Indication: schizophrenia (schizophrénie)

Pulmonary Medications

Flovent Inhalation Aerosol
    Generic/Dose: fluticasone propionate (fluticason proprionate)
                110 mcg/spray and 220 mcg/spray
    Indication: asthma (asthme)

Flovent Rotadisk
  Generic/Dose: fluticasone propionate inhalation powder (fluticas
              on proprionate) 50 mcg/dose, 100 mcg/dose, 250
              mcg/dose
  Indication: asthma (asthme)

Atrovent
  Generic/Dose: ipratropium bromide (ipratropium bromure mono
              hydrate) 18 mcg/inhalation
  Indication: asthma (asthme)

Atrovent Nasal Spray
  Generic/Dose: ipratropium bromide (ipratropium bromure mono
              hydrate) 0.03% and 0.06%
  Indication: asthma (asthme)

Singulair
  Generic/Dose: montelukast (montélukast sel de Na) 5 mg, 10 mg
  Indication: asthma (asthme)

Vancenase AQ DS
  Generic/Dose: beclamethasone dipropionate (béclométasone
              diproprionate) 84 mcg/spray
  Indication: asthma (asthme)

Azmacort
  Generic/Dose: triamcinolone acetonide (triamcinolone acétonide)
              1, 2, 4, 8 mg tablets.
  Indication: asthma (asthme)

Combivent (Ipratropium/albuterol)
  Generic/Dose: ipratropium bromide (ipratropium bromure mono
              hydrate) 21 mcg abuterol sulfate (salbutamol
              sulfate) 120 mcg
  Indication: bronchospasm (bronchospasme)

Proventil
  Generic/Dose: albuterol (salbutamol sulfate) 90 mcg/spray
  Indication: bronchospasm (bronchospasme)

Serevent
   Generic/Dose: salmeterol (salmeterol) 21 mcg/spray
   Indication: asthma (asthme)

Urologic Medications

Viagra
   Generic/Dose: sidenafil citrate (sildenafil citrate) 25 mg, 50 mg,
                 100 mg
   Indication: impotence (impuissance)

Cardura
   Generic/Dose: doxazosin (doxazosin mésilate) 1 mg, 2 mg, 4 mg,
                 8 mg
   Indication: benign prostate hypertrophy (hypertrophie de la
                 prostate)
                 hypertension (hypertension)

Detrol
   Generic/Dose: tolterodine (toltérodine L–tartrate) 1 mg, 2 mg
   Indication: urinary incontinence (incontinence d'urine)

Hytrin
   Generic/Dose: terazosin (térazosine chlorhydrate dihydraté) 1 mg,
                 2 mg, 5 mg , 10 mg
   Indication: benign prostatic hypertrophy (hypertrophie de la
                 prostate)
                 hypertension (hypertension)

Flomax (tamsulosin)
   Generic/Dose: tamsulosin (tamsulosine chlorhydrate) 0.4 mg
   Indication: urinary retention (rétention d'urine)

Non-Prescription Medications

The non-prescription medication section is designed to assist you in identifying over-the-counter (OTC) medications that you may need during your travels. The list represents selections from over 350 available medications. Many medications have variations. Due to size constraints, the list has been reduced to those that will provide relief for a broad number of conditions.

The most effective way to use this section is to review your needs (cough, sinusitis, congestion, etc.) and select the appropriate medications. A translation of the generic medication and the dose are provided when available. The pharmacist should be able to select a comparable medication. Please note that the pharmaceutical industry changes rapidly. Many efforts have been made to ensure the accuracy of the data. All doses are listed per tablet, unless otherwise specified.

Always fill out your Medical History Section, Allergy Section, and Medications first. This provides invaluable information for those trying to assist you. Remember, the more information you can provide, the better your choices. Communication of this type can take time. Foreign health care professionals are there to assist you. Do not rush them.

Conversions
1 teaspoon = 5 milliliters (ml)
1 tablespoon = 15 milliliters (ml)
1 dropperful = 0.8 milliliters (ml)

Adult Medications

Antihistamines, Analgesics, Colds, Cough, Congestion, Sore Throat, etc.
The following is a list of medications that should be able to provide some relief. This is only a partial list of medications available in the United States. It will provide useful information for the most frequent outpatient problem: the common cold. After each medication, a list of specific complaints treated by the drug is listed.

Chlorpheniramine maleate (chlorphénanamine maleáte): a
  sedating antihistamine

Pseudoephedrine (pseudoéphédrine): nasal decongestant
Dextromethorphan (dextrométhorphane): cough suppressant for
non-productive (dry) cough
Doxylamine succinate (doxylamine): sedating antihistamine
Guaifenesin (guaïfénésine): expectorant for productive cough

Abreva
Generic/Dose: docosanol 10% cream
Indication: oral cold sore
herpes virus (hèrpes virus)

Aleve
Generic/Dose: naproxen sodium (naproxéne sel de Na) 220 mg
Indication: analgesic (analgésique)

Aleve Cold and Sinus
Generic/Dose: naproxen sodium (naproxéne sel de Na) 220 mg
pseudoephedrine HCL (pseudoéphédrine
chlorhy drate) 120 mg
Indication: analgesic (analgésique)
decongestant (décongestant)

Alka-Seltzer
Generic/Dose: aspirin (acid acétylsalicylique) 325 mg, citric acid
(citrate disodique anydre) 1000 mg, sodium bicarbonate (carbonate monosodique) 1916 mg
Indication: analgesic (analgésique)

Alka-Seltzer Extra Strength
Generic/Dose: aspirin (acid acétylsalicylique) 500 mg, citric acid
(citrate disodique anydre) 1000 mg, sodium bicarbonate (carbonate monosodique) 1916 mg
Indication: analgesic (analgésique)

Alka-Seltzer PM
Generic/Dose: aspirin (acid acétylsalicylique) 325 mg,
diphenhydramine citrate (diphéhydramine chlorh-
drate) 38 mg

Indication: analgesic (analgésique)
                insomnia (insomnie)

Alka-Seltzer Heartburn Relief
Generic/Dose: citric acid (citrate disodique anhydre) 1000 mg,
                sodium bicarbonate (carbonate monosodique)
                1940 mg
Indication: indigestion (dyspepsie)

Alka-Seltzer Plus Cold Medicine
Generic/Dose: acetaminophen (paracétamol) 325 mg
                chlorpheniramine maleate (chlorphénanamine
                    maleáte) 2 mg
                pseudoephedrine hydrochloride
                    (pseudoéphédrine chlorhydrate) 30 mg
Indication: analgesic (analgésique)
                decongestant (décongestant)

Alka-Seltzer Plus Cough and Cold
Generic/Dose: acetaminophen (paracétamol) 325 mg
                dextromethorphan hydrobromide (dextrométhor
                    phanebromhydrate) 10 mg
                doxylamine succinate (doxylamine succinate)
                    6.25 mg
                pseudoephedrine hydrochloride (pseudoéphédrine
                    chlorhydrate) 30 mg
                chlorpheniramine maleate (chlorphénanamine
                    maleáte) 2 mg
Indication: analgesic (analgésique)
                decongestant (décongestant)

Alka-Seltzer Plus Cold and Flu
Generic/Dose: acetaminophen (paracétamol) 325 mg
                dextromethorphan hydrobromide (dextrométhor-
                phane bromhydrate) 10 mg
                pseudoephedrine hydrochloride (pseudoéphédrine
                chlorhydrate) 30 mg
Indication: analgesic (analgésique)
                decongestant (décongestant)

Alka-Seltzer Plus Cold and Sinus
   Generic/Dose: acetaminophen (paracétamol) 325 mg
               pseudoephedrine-hydrochloride (pseudoéphédrine
               chlorhydrate) 30 mg
   Indication: analgesic (analgésique)
               decongestant (décongestant)

Alka-Seltzer Plus Nighttime Cold Medicine
   Generic/Dose: acetaminophen (paracétamol) 325 mg
               dextromethorphan hydrobromide (dextrométhor-
               phane bromhydrate) 10 mg
               doxylamine succinate (doxylamine succinate) 6.25
               mg
               pseudoephedrine hydrochloride (pseudoéphédrine
               chlorhydrate) 30 mg
   Indication: analgesic (analgésique)
               insomnia (insomnie)
               decongestant (décongestant)

Bengay Arthritis Cream
   Generic/Dose: methyl salicylate (salicylate de méthyl) 18.3%
               menthol (menthol) 16%
   Indication: arthritis (arthrite)
               analgesic (analgésique)

Bayer Aspirin
   Generic/Dose: aspirin (acid acétylsalicylique) 325 mg
   Indication: analgesic (analgésique)

Bayer Extra Strength Plus
   Generic/Dose: aspirin (acid acétylsalicylique) 500 mg calcium
               carbonate (calcium carbonate)
   Indication: analgesic (analgésique)
               buffered preparation

Bayer Extra Strength PM
   Generic/Dose: aspirin (acid acétylsalicylique) 500 mg
               diphenhydramine hydrochloride (diphéhydramine

chlorhydrate) 25 mg
Indication: analgesic (analgésique)
                insomnia (insomnie)

Natruvent Nasal Saline Spray
   Generic/Dose: oxylometazoline hydrochloride (oxymétazoline
                chlorhydrate) 0.1%
   Indication: decongestant (décongestant)

Comtrex Mulitsystem Cold & Cough Relief
   Generic/Dose: acetaminophen (paracétamol) 500 mg
                pseudoephedrine hydrochloride (psudoéphédrine
                chlorhydrate) 30 mg
                chlorpheniramine maleate (chlorphénanamine
                maleáte) 2 mg
                dextromethorphan hydrobromide (dextrométhor-
                phane bromhydrate) 15 mg
   Indication: analgesic (analgésique)
                decongestant (décongestant)

Comtrex Deep Chest Cold & Congestion Relief
   Generic/Dose: acetaminophen (paracétamol) 250 mg
                dextromethorphan hydrobromide (dextrométhor-
                phane bromhydrate) 10 mg
                guaifenesin (guaïfénésine) 100 mg
                pseudoephedrine hydrochloride (psudoéphédrine
                chlorhydrate) 30 mg
   Indication: analgesic (analgésique)
                decongestant (décongestant)

Comtrex Acute Head Cold & Sinus Pressure Relief
   Generic/Dose: acetaminophen (paracétamol) 500 mg
                pseudoephedrine hydrochloride (psudoéphédrine
                chlorhydrate) 30 mg
                brompheniramine maleate (bromphéniramine
                maléate) 2 mg
   Indication: analgesic (analgésique)
                decongestant (décongestant)

Excedrin PM
  Generic/Dose: acetaminophen (paracétamol) 250 mg
                diphenhydramine citrate (diphenhydramine chlorhy-
                drate) 38 mg
  Indication: analgesic (analgésique)
                insomnia (insomnie)

Primatene Mist
  Generic/Dose: epinephrine (epinephrine) 0.22 mg/inhalation
                (5.5 mg/ml epinephrine)
  Indication: asthma (asthma)

Excedrin Aspirin Free
  Generic/Dose: acetaminophen (paracétamol) 500 mg caffeine
                (caféine) 65 mg
  Indication: analgesic (analgésique)

Excedrin Extra Strength
  Generic/Dose: acetaminophen (paracétamol) 250 mg aspirin (acid
                acétylsalicylique) 250 mg caffeine (caféine) 65 mg
  Indication: analgesic (analgésique)

Tylenol Extra Strength
  Generic/Dose: acetaminophen (paracétamol) 500 mg
  Indication: analgesic (analgésique)

Tylenol Regular Strength
  Generic/Dose: acetaminophen (paracétamol) 325 mg
  Indication: analgesic (analgésique)

Tylenol Maximum Strength Allergy and Sinus
  Generic/Dose: acetaminophen (paracétamol) 500 mg
                chlorpheniramine maleate (chlorphénanamine
                maleáte) 2 mg
                pseudoephedrine hydrochloride (pséudoephédrine
                chlorhydrate) 30 mg
  Indication: analgesic (analgésique)
                decongestant (décongestant)

Tylenol Severe Allergy
    Generic/Dose: acetaminophen (paracétamol) 500 mg
                diphenhydramine hydrochloride (diphénhydramine
                chlorhydrate) 12.5 mg
    Indication: analgesic (analgésique)
                decongestant (décongestant)

Tylenol Arthritis Pain Extended Relief
    Generic/Dose: acetaminophen (paracétamol) 650 mg
    Indication: analgesic (analgésique)
                extended relief

Tylenol Multi Symptom Cold Complete Formula
    Generic/Dose: acetaminophen (paracétamol) 325 mg
                chlorpheniramine maleate (chlorphéniramine
                maleáte) 2 mg
                dextromethorphan hydrobromide (dextrométhor-
                phane bromhydrate) 15 mg
                pseudoephedrine hydrochloride (pseudoéphédrine
                chlorhydrate) 30 mg
    Indication: analgesic (analgésique)
                decongestant (décongestant)

Tylenol Multi-Symptom Cold Non-Drowsy
    Generic/Dose: acetaminophen (paracétamol) 325 mg
                dextromethorphan hydrobromide (dextrométhor-
                phane bromhydrate) 15 mg
                pseudoephedrine hydrochloride (pseudoéphédrine
                chlorhydrate) 30 mg
    Indication: analgesic (analgésique)

Tylenol Cold Severe Congestion Non-Drowsy
    Generic/Dose: acetaminophen (paracétamol) 325 mg
                dextromethorphan hydrobromide (dextrométhor-
                phane bromhydrate) 15 mg
                guaifenesin (guaïfénésine) 200 mg
                pseudoephedrine hydrochloride (pseudoéphédrine
                chlorhydrate) 30 mg

Indication: analgesic (analgésique)
                decongestant (décongestant)

Tylenol Maximum Strength Flu Nighttime
  Generic/Dose: acetaminophen (paracétamol) 500 mg
                diphenhydramine hydrochloride (diphénhydramine
                chlorhydrate) 25 mg
                pseudoephedrine hydrochloride (pseudoéphédrine
                chlorhydrate) 30 mg
  Indication: analgesic (analgésique)
                decongestant (décongestant)
                insomnia (insomnie)

Tylenol Maximum Strength Flu Nighttime Liquid (per 30 ml or
                2 tbsp.)
  Generic/Dose: acetaminophen (paracétamol) 1000 mg
                dextromethorphan hydrobromide (dextrométhor-
                phane bromhydrate) 30 mg
                doxylamine succinate (doxylamine succinate)
                12.5 mg
                pseudoephedrine hydrochloride (pseudoéphédrine
                chlorhydrate) 60 mg
  Indication: analgesic (analgésique)
                decongestant (décongestant)
                insomnia (insomnie)
                elixir (élixir)

Tylenol Maximum Strength Flu Non-Drowsy
  Generic/Dose: acetaminophen (paracétamol) 500 mg
                dextromethorphan hydrobromide (dextrométhor-
                phane bromhydrate) 15 mg
                pseudoephedrine hydrochloride (pseudoéphédrine
                chlorhydrate) 30 mg
  Indication: analgesic (analgésique)
                decongestant (décongestant)

Tylenol Extra Strength PM
  Generic/Dose: acetaminophen (paracétamol) 500 mg

diphenhydramine hydrochloride (diphénhydramine chlorhydrate) 25 mg
Indication: analgesic (analgésique)
insomnia (insomnie)

Tylenol Maximum Strength Sinus Nighttime Caplets
Generic/Dose: acetaminophen (paracétamol) 500 mg
doxylamine succinate (doxylamine succinate) 6.25 mg
pseudoephedrine hydrochloride (pseudoéphédrine chlorhydrate) 30 mg
Indication: analgesic (analgésique)
decongestant (décongestant)
insomnia (insomnie)

Tylenol Maximum Strength Sinus Non Drowsy
Generic/Dose: acetaminophen (paracétamol) 500 mg
pseudoephedrine hydrochloride (pseudoéphédrine chlorhydrate) 30 mg
Indication: analgesic (analgésique)
decongestant (décongestant)

Tylenol Maximum Strength Sore Throat Liquid
Generic/Dose: acetaminophen (paracétamol) 100 mg/30 ml
Indication: analgesic (analgésique)

Tylenol Maximum Strength Multi-Symptom Menstrual Relief
Generic/Dose: acetaminophen (paracétamol) 500 mg
pamabrom 25 mg
Indication: analgesic (analgésique)
menstruation (menstruation)

Delsym Cough Formula
Generic/Dose: dextromethorphan polistirex (dextrométhorphane bromhydrate) 30mg/5ml
Indication: antitussive (expectorant)
extended release formula

Tavist Allergy
  Generic/Dose: clemastine fumarate USP 1.34 mg
  Indication: decongestant (décongestant)
                 antihistamine

Tavist Sinus Non Drowsy
  Generic/Dose: acetaminophen (paracétamol) 500 mg
                 pseudoephedrine hydrochloride (pseudoéphédrine
                 chlorhydrate) 30 mg
  Indication: analgesic (analgésique)
                 decongestant (décongestant)

TheraFlu Maximum Strength Flu and Congestion Non-Drowsy
                 (doses are per packet)
  Generic/Dose: acetaminophen (paracétamol) 1000 mg
                 guaifenesin (guaïfénésine) 400 mg
                 pseudoephedrine hydrochloride (pseudoéphédrine
                 chlorhydrate) 60 mg
                 dextromethorphan hydrobromide (dextrométhor-
                 phane bromhydrate) 30 mg
  Indication: decongestant (décongestant)
                 analgesic (analgésique)

TheraFlu Maximum Strength Flu & Cough Night Time (doses are
                 per packet)
  Generic/Dose: acetaminophen (paracétamol) 1000 mg
                 pseudoephedrine hydrochloride (pseudoéphédrine
                 chlorhydrate) 60 mg
                 dextromethorphan hydrobromide (dextrométhor-
                 phane bromhydrate) 30 mg
                 chlorpheniramine maleate (chlorphénanamine
                 maleáte) 4 mg
  Indication: analgesic (analgésique)
                 decongestant (décongestant)

TheraFlu Maximum Strength Sever Cold and Congestion
                 Non-Drowsy

Generic/Dose: acetaminophen (paracétamol) 1000 mg.
pseudoephedrine hydrochloride (peudoéphédrine chlorhydrate) 60 mg
dextromethorphan hydrobromide (dextrométhorphane bromhydrate) 30 mg
Indication: analgesic (analgésique)
decongestant (décongestant)

TheraFlu Regular Strength Cold & Sore Throat Night Time
(doses per packet)
Generic/Dose: acetaminophen (paracétamol) 650 mg
pseudoephedrine hydrochloride (peudoéphédrine chlorhydrate) 60 mg
chlorpheniramine maleate (chlorphénanamine maleáte) 4 mg
Indication: analgesic (analgésique)
decongestant (décongestant)

Triaminic Allergy Congestion
Generic/Dose: pseudoephedrine hydrochloride (peudoéphédrine chlorhydrate) 15 mg/5 ml
Indication: decongestant (décongestant)

Triaminic Chest Congestion Expectorant, Nasal Decongestant
Generic/Dose: guaifenesin (guaïfénésine) USP 50 mg/5 ml
pseudoephedrine hydrochloride (peudoéphédrine chlorhydrate) 15 mg/5 ml
Indication: expectorant (expectorant)
decongestant (décongestant)

Triaminic Cold & Allergy, Nasal Decongestant, Antihistamine
Generic/Dose: pseudoephedrine hydrochloride (peudoéphédrine chlorhydrate) 50 mg/5 ml
chlorpheniramine maleate (chlorphénanamine maleáte) 1 mg/5 ml
Indication: decongestant (décongestant)

Triaminic Cough & Cold
Generic/Dose: pseudoephedrine hydrochloride (peudoéphédrine
        chlorhydrate) 15 mg
        dextromethorphan hydrobromide (dextrométhor-
        phane bromhydrate) 5 mg
        chlorpheniramine maleate (chlorphénanamine
        maleáte) 1 mg
Indication: decongestant (décongestant)
        antitussive (expectorant)

Triaminic Cold, Cough & Fever
Generic/Dose: acetaminophen (paracétamol) 160 mg/5 ml
        pseudoephedrine hydrochloride (peudoéphédrine
        chlorhydrate) 15 mg/5 ml
        dextromethorphan hydrobromide (dextrométhor-
        phane bromhydrate) 7.5 mg/5 ml
        chlorpheniramine maleate (chlorphénanamine
        maleáte) 1 mg/5 ml
Indication: analgesic (analgésique)
        decongestant (décongestant)
        antitussive (expectorant)

Triaminic Cold & Night Time Cough
Generic/Dose: pseudoephedrine hypochlorite (peudoéphédrine
        chlorhydrate) 15 mg
        dextromethorphan hydrobromide (dextrométhor-
        phane bromhydrate) 7.5 mg
        chlorpheniramine maleate (chlorphénanamine
        maleáte) 1.0 mg
Indication: analgesic (analgésique)
        decongestant (décongestant)
        antitussive (expectorant)

Triaminic Cough
Generic/Dose: pseudoephedrine hydrochloride (peudoéphédrine
        chlorhydrate) 15 mg/5 ml
        dextromethorphan hydrobromide (dextrométhor-

phane bromhydrate) 5 mg/5 ml
Indication: antitussive (expectorant)

Triaminic Cough & Congestion
Generic/Dose: pseudoephedrine hydrochloride (peudoéphédrine
                chlorhydrate) 15 mg
                dextromethorphan hydrobromide (dextrométhor-
                phane bromhydrate) 7.5 mg
Indication: decongestant (décongestant)
                antitussive (expectorant)

Triaminic Cough & Sore Throat
Generic/Dose: acetaminophen (paracétamol) 160 mg/5 ml
                pseudoephedrine hydrochloride (peudoéphédrine
                chlorhydrate) 15 mg/5 ml
                dextromethorphan hydrobromide (dextrométhor-
                phane bromhydrate) 7.5 mg/5 ml
Indication: analgesic (analgésique)
                decongestant (décongestant)

Actifed Cold & Allergy
Generic/Dose: pseudoephedrine hydrochloride
                (peudoéphédrine chlorhydrate) 60 mg
                triprolidine hydrochloride (triprolidine chlorhy-
                drate) 2.5 mg
Indication: decongestant (décongestant)

Actifed Cold & Sinus
Generic/Dose: acetaminophen (paracétamol) 500 mg
                pseudoephedrine hydrochloride (pseudoéphédrine
                chlorhydrate) 30 mg
                chlorpheniramine maleate (chlorphénanamine
                maleáte) 2 mg
Indication: analgesic (analgésique)
                decongestant (décongestant)

Benadryl Allergy Chewable Tablets
Generic/Dose: diphenhydramine 12.5 mg
Indication: allergy relief

Benadryl Allergy Liquid Medication
  Generic/Dose: diphenhydramine hydrochloride (diphénhydramine
          chlorhydrate) 12.5 mg/5 ml
  Indication: allergy relief
          elixir (élixir)

Benadryl Allergy/Cold Tablets
  Generic/Dose: diphenhydramine hydrochloride (diphénhydramine
          chlorhydrate) 12.5 mg
          pseudoephedrine hydrochloride (pseudoéphédrine
          chlorhydrate) 30 mg
          acetaminophen (paracétamol) 500 mg
  Indication: allergy relief
          decongestant (décongestant)
          analgesic (analgésique)

Benadryl Allergy/Congestion Tablets
  Generic/Dose: diphenhydramine hydrochloride (diphénhydramine
          chlorhydrate) 25 mg
          pseudoephedrine hydrochloride (pseudoéphédrine
          chlorhydrate) 60 mg
  Indication: allergy relief
          decongestant (décongestant)

Benadryl Dye-Free Allergy Liquid Medication
  Generic/Dose: diphenhydramine hydrochloride (diphénhy-
          dramine) 12.5 mg/5 ml
  Indication: allergy relief
          dye free

Benadryl Allergy/Sinus Headache Tablets
  Generic/Dose: diphenhydramine hydrochloride (diphénhydramine
          chlorhydrate) 12.5 mg
          pseudoephedrine hydrochloride (pseudoéphédrine
          chlorhydrate) 30 mg
          acetaminophen (paracétamol) 500 mg
  Indication: allergy relief
          decongestant (décongestant)
          analgesic (analgésique)

Benadryl Severe Allergy and Sinus Headache Maximum Strength
Generic/Dose: diphenhydramine hydrochloride (diphénhydramine
chlorhydrate) 25 mg
pseudoephedrine hydrochloride (pseudoéphédrine
chlorhydrate) 30 mg
acetaminophen (paracétamol) 500 mg
Indication: analgesic (analgésique)
decongestant (décongestant)

Benylin Adult Cough Suppressant
Generic/Dose: dextromethorphan hydrobromide (dextrométhor-
phane bromhydrate) 15 mg
Indication: antitussive (expectorant)

Benylin Multi-Symptom Cough
Generic/Dose: guaifenesin (guaïfénésine) 100 mg/5 ml
pseudoephedrine hydrochloride (pseudoéphédrine
chlorhydrate) 50 mg/5 ml
dextromethorphan hydrobromide (dextrométho-r
phane bromhydrate) 5 mg/5 ml
Indication: antitussive (expectorant)
decongestant (décongestant)

Sinutab Non Drying Liquid Caps
Generic/Dose: pseudoephedrine hydrochloride (pseudoéphédrine
chlorhydrate) 30 mg
guaifenesin (guaïfénésine) 200 mg
Indication: allergy relief
decongestant (décongestant)

Sinutab Sinus Allergy Maximum Strength
Generic/Dose: acetaminophen (paracétamol) 5 mg
chlorpheniramine maleate (chlorphénanamine
maleáte) 2 mg
pseudoephedrine hydrochloride (pseudoéphédrine
chlorhydrate) 30 mg
Indication: allergy relief
analgesic (analgésique)
decongestant (décongestant)

Sudafed Cold and Allergy
Generic/Dose: chlorpheniramine maleate (chlorphenanamine
maleate) 4 mg
pseudoephedrine hydrochloride (pseudoéphédrine
chlorhydrate) 60 mg
Indication: allergy relief
decongestant (décongestant)

Sudafed Cold and Cough Liquid Caplets (dose/liquid caplets)
Generic/Dose: acetaminophen (paracétamol) 250 mg
guaifenesin (guaïfénésine) 100 mg
pseudoephedrine hydrochloride (pseudoéphédrine
chlorhydrate) 30 mg
dextromethorphan hydrochloride (dextrométhorphane chlorhydrate) 10 mg
Indication: analgesic (analgésique)
decongestant (décongestant)
antitussive (expectorant)

Sudafed Cold and Sinus Liquid Caps
Generic/Dose: acetaminophen (paracétamol) 325 mg
pseudoephedrine hydrochloride (pseudoéphédrine
chlorhydrate) 30 mg
Indication: analgesic (analgésique)
decongestant (décongestant)

Sudafed Severe Cold Formula
Generic/Dose: acetaminophen (paracétamol) 500 mg
pseudoephedrine hydrochloride (pseudoéphédrine
bromhydrate) 30 mg
dextromethorphan hydrobromide (dextrométhorphane bromhydrate) 15 mg
Indication: analgesic (analgésique)
decongestant (décongestant)

Sudafed 12 hour
Generic/Dose: pseudoephedrine hydrochloride (pseudoéphédrine
chlorhydrate) 120 mg
Indication: decongestant (décongestant)
extended release formulation

Sudafed 24 hour
  Generic/Dose: pseudoephedrine hydrochloride (pseudoéphédrine
               chlorhydrate) 240 mg
               (80 mg immediate release, 160 mg extended
               release)
  Indication: decongestant (décongestant)
               extended release formulation

Vicks 44 Cough Relief
  Generic/Dose: dextromethorphan hydrobromide (dextrométhor-
               phane bromhydrate) 30 mg/15 ml
  Indication: antitussive (expectorant)

Vicks 44 D
  Generic/Dose: dextromethorphan hydrobromide (dextrométhor-
               phane bromhydrate) 30 mg/15 ml
               pseudoephedrine hydrochloride 60 mg/15 ml
  Indication: antitussive (expectorant)
               decongestant (décongestant)

Vicks 44 E
  Generic/Dose: dextromethorphan hydrobromide (dextrométhor-
               phane bromhydrate) 20 mg/15 ml
               guaifenesin (guaïfénésine) 200 mg/15 ml
  Indication: antitussive (expectorant)
               decongestant (décongestant)
               expectorant (expectorant)

Vicks 44 M Cough, Cold & Flu Relief Liquid
  Generic/Dose: dextromethorphan hydrobromide (dextrométhor-
               phane bromhydrate) 30 mg/20 ml
               pseudoephedrine hydrochloride (pseudoéphédrine
               chlorhydrate) 60 mg/20 ml
               chlorpheniramine maleate (chlorphénanamine
               maleáte) 4 mg/20 ml
               acetaminophen (paracétamol) 650 mg/20 ml
  Indication: decongestant (décongestant)
               antitussive (expectorant)
               elixir (élixir)

Afrin Original 12 Hour Nasal Spray
Generic/Dose: oxymetazoline (oxymétazoline) articled 0.05%
Indication: decongestant (décongestant)
              nasal spray

Chlor-Trimeton Allergy (12 hour)
Generic/Dose: chlorpheniramine maleate (chlorphéniramine
              maleáte) 12 mg
Indication: allergy relief
              extended release

Chlor-Trimeton Allergy D (12 hour)
Generic/Dose: chlorpheniramine maleate (chlorphéniramine pseu-
              doephedrine hydrochloride (pseudoéphédrine
              chlorhydrate) 120 mg
Indication: decongestant (décongestant)
              allergy relief
              extended release

Coricidin D
Generic/Dose: acetaminophen (paracétamol) 325 mg
              chlorpheniramine maleate (chlorphéniramine
              maleáte) 2 mg
              pseudoephedrine hydrochloride (pseudoéphédrine
              chlorhydrate) 30 mg
Indication: analgesic (analgésique)
              decongestant (décongestant)

Coricidin HBP Cough and Cold Relief
Generic/Dose: acetominophen (paracétamol) 325 mg
              chlorpheniramine maleate (chlorphéniramine
              maleáte) 2 mg
Indication: antitussive (expectorant)
              For patients with hypertension

Coricidin HBP Cold and Flu Relief
Generic/Dose: chlorpheniramine maleate (chlorphéniramine
              maleáte) 4 mg
              dextromethorphan hydrobromide (dextrométhor-
              phane bromhydrate) 30 mg

Indication: decongestant (décongestant)
                For patients with hypertension

Coricidin HBP Night Time Cold and Flu Relief
Generic/Dose: acetaminophen (paracétamol) 325 mg
                diphenhydramine hydrochloride (diphénhydramine
                chlorhydrate) 25 mg
Indication: analgesic (analgésique)
                decongestant (décongestant)
                For patients with hypertension

Coricidin HBP Maximum Strength Flu Relief
Generic/Dose: acetaminophen (paracétamol) 500 mg
                chlorpheniramine maleate (chlorphéniramine
                maleáte) 2 mg
                dextromethorphan hydrobromide (dextrométhor-
                phane bromhydrate) 15 mg
Indication: analgesic (analgésique)
                decongestant (décongestant)
                For patients with hypertension

Drixoral Cold & Allergy Sustained Action Tablets
Generic/Dose: pseudoephedrine sulfate (pseudophephedrine
                sulfate) 120 mg
                dexbrompheniramine maleate 6 mg
Indication: allergy relief
                decongestant (décongestant)
                extended release formulation

Drixoral Allergy & Sinus
Generic/Dose: pseudoephedrine sulfate (pseudoéphédrine sulfate)
                60 mg
                dexbrompheniramine maleate 3 mg
                acetaminophen (paracétamol) 500 mg
Indication: allergy relief
                decongestant (décongestant)
                analgesic (analgésique)

Drixoral Cold & Flu (time released preparation)
  Generic/Dose: acetaminophen (paracétamol) 500 mg
              dexbrompheniramine maleate 3 mg
              pseudoephedrine sulfate (pseudoéphédrine sulfate)
                60 mg
  Indication: analgesic (analgésique)
              extended release formula

Drixoral Nasal Decongestant
  Generic/Dose: pseudoephedrine sulfate (pseudoéphédrine sulfate)
                120 mg
  Indication: decongestant (décongestant)
              extended release formula

Contac Non-Drowsy 12 Hour Cold Caplets
  Generic/Dose: pseudoephedrine hydrochloride (pseudoéphédrine
              chlorhydrate) 120 mg
  Indication: decongestant (décongestant)
              extended release

Contac Maximum Strength Severe Cold & Flu
  Generic/Dose: acetaminophen (paracétamol) 500 mg
              pseudoephedrine hydrochloride (pseudoéphédrine
              chlorhydrate) 30 mg
              dextromethorphan hydrobromide (dextromethor-
              phane bromhydrate) 15 mg
              chlorpheniramine maleate (chlorphénanamine
              maleáte) 2 mg
  Indication: analgesic (analgésique)
              decongestant (décongestant)
              antitussive (expectorant)

Advil
  Generic/Dose: ibuprofen (ibuproféne) 200 mg
  Indication: analgesic (analgésique)

Advil Cold & Sinus
  Generic/Dose: ibuprofen (ibuproféne) 200 mg

pseudoephedrine hydrochloride 30 mg
Indication: analgesic (analgésique)
decongestant (décongestant)

Dimetapp Cold & Fever Suspension
Generic/Dose: acetaminophen (paracétamol) 160 mg/5 ml
bromphéniramine maleate (brompheniramine
maléate) 1 mg/5 ml
pseudoephedrine hydrochloride (pseudoéphédrine
chlorhydrate) 15 mg/5 ml
Indication: analgesic (analgésique)
decongestant (décongestant)

Dimetapp DM Cold & Cough Elixir
Generic/Dose: brompheniramine maleate (brompheniramine
maleate) 1 mg/5 ml
pseudoephedrine hydrochloride (pseudoéphédrine
chlorhydrate) 50 mg/5 ml
dextromethorphan hydrobromide (dextrométhorphane bromhydrate) 5 mg/5 ml
Indication: antitussive (expectorant)
decongestant (décongestant)
elixir (élixir)

Dimetapp Nighttime Flu Syrup
Generic/Dose: acetaminophen (paracétamol) 160 mg/5 ml
brompheniramine maleate (bromphéniramine
maléate) 1 mg/5 ml
dextromethorphan hydrobromide (dextrométhorphane bromhydrate) 5 mg/5 ml
pseudoephedrine hydrochloride (pseudoéphédrine
chlorhydrate) 15 mg/5 ml
Indication: analgesic (analgésique)
decongestant (décongestant)
antitussive (expectorant)

Dimetapp Non-Drowsy Flu Syrup
Generic/Dose: acetaminophen (paracétamol) 160 mg/5 ml

dextromethorphan hydrobromide (dextrométhorphane bromhydrate) 5 mg/5 ml
pseudoephedrine hydrochloride (pseudoéphédrine chlorhydrate) 15 mg/5 ml
Indication: analgesic (analgésique)
decongestant (décongestant)

Dimetapp Elixir
Generic/Dose: brompheniramine maleate (bromphéniramine maléate) 1 mg/5 ml
pseudoephedrine hydrochloride (pseudoéphédrine chlorhydrate) 15 mg/5 ml
Indication: decongestant (décongestant)
antihistamine
elixir (élixir)

Robitussin Cold Multi System Cold and Flu Softgels
Generic/Dose: acetaminophen (paracétamol) 200 mg
guaifenesin (guaïfénésine) 100 mg
pseudoephedrine hydrochloride (pseudoéphédrine chlorhydrate) 30 mg
dextromethorphan hydrobromide (dextromethorphane bromhydrate) 10 mg
Indication: analgesic (analgésique)
decongestant (décongestant)
Wantitussive (expectorant)

Robitussin Cough Drops
Generic/Dose: menthol (menthol) 10 mg
Indication: antitussive (expectorant)

Robitussin PE Syrup
Generic/Dose: guaifenesin (guaïfénésine) 100 mg/5 ml
pseudoephedrine hydrochloride (pseudoéphédrine chlorhydrate) 30 mg/5 ml
Indication: antitussive (expectorant)

Robitussin Maximum Strength Cough & Cold Elixir
Generic/Dose: dextromethorphan hydrobromide (dextromethor
     phane bromhydrate) 15 mg/5 ml
     pseudoephedrine hydrochloride (pseudoéphédrine
     chlorhydrate) 30 mg/5 ml
Indication: antitussive (expectorant)
     decongestant (décongestant)

Cepacol Maximum Strength Sore Throat Lozenges
Generic/Dose: menthol (menthol) 2 mg
Indication: lozenges (pastille)

Cepacol Viractin Cold Sore Treatment
Generic/Dose: tetracaine (tetracaïne chlorhydrate) 2%
Indication: oral analgesic (analgésique)
     topical medication

Neo-Synephrine
Generic/Dose: oxymetazoline hydrochloride (oxymétazoline
     chlorhydrate) 0.05%
Indication: nasal spray decongestant (decongestant)

Vanquish Extra Strength Pain Formula
Generic/Dose: aspirin (acid acétylsalicylique) 227 mg
     acetaminophen (paracétamol) 194 mg
     caffeine (caféine) 33 mg
Indication: analgesic (analgésique)

Vanquish Extra Strength Pain Formula With Buffers
Generic/Dose: aspirin (acid acétylsalicylique) 227 mg
     acetaminophen (paracétamol) 194 mg
     caffeine (caféine) 33 mg
     aluminum hydroxide (aluminum hydroxyde)
     magnesium hydroxide (magnésium hyrdroxyde)
Indication: analgesic (analgésique)

Motrin Migraine Pain
Generic/Dose: ibuprofen (ibuproféne) 200 mg

Indication: analgesic (analgésique)
                migraine headaches (migraine)

Motrin IB
  Generic/Dose: ibuprofen (ibuproféne) 200 mg
  Indication: analgesic (analgésique)

Motrin Sinus Headache
  Generic/Dose: ibuprofen (ibuproféne) 200 mg
                pseudoephedrine hydrochloride (pseudoéphédrine chlorhydrate) 30 mg
  Indication: analgesic (analgésique)
                decongestant (décongestant)

Emetrol
  Generic/Dose: dextrose 1.87 g/5 ml
                fructose (fructose) 1.87 g/5 ml
                phosphoric acid 21.5 mg/5 ml
  Indication: nausea (nausée)
                vomiting (vomissement)

Zilactin
  Generic/Dose: benzyl alcohol 10%
  Indication: analgesic (analgésique)

Percogesic
  Generic/Dose: acetaminophen (paracétamol) 500 mg
                diphenhydramine hydrochloride (diphénhydramine chlorhydrate) 12.5 mg
  Indication: analgesic (analgésique)

NasalCrom Nasal Spray
  Generic/Dose: cromolyn sodium 40 mg/ml
  Indication: rhinitis (rhinite)

Ecotrin Low Strength Aspirin
  Generic/Dose: aspirin (acid acetylsalicylique) 81 mg
  Indication: analgesic (analgésique)

Ecotrin Regular Strength Aspirin
   Generic/Dose: aspirin (acid acetylsalicylique) 325 mg
   Indication: analgesic (analgésique)

Ecotrin Maximum Strength Aspirin
   Generic/Dose: aspirin (acid acetylsalicylique) 500 mg
   Indication: analgesic (analgésique)

Abdominal Pain, Heartburn, Constipation, Diarrhea, and Mouth Care

Phillips Fiber Caps
   Generic/Dose: calcium carbophil 625 mg
   Indication: constipation (constipation)

Phillips Milk of Magnesia
   Generic/Dose: magnesium hydroxide (magnésium hyrdroxyde)
               400 mg/5 ml
   Indication: constipation (constipation)

Natural relief of constipation
   Generic/Dose: senna (séné) 8.6 mg
   Indication: constipation (constipation)

Regular Strength Mylanta
   Generic/Dose: aluminum hydroxide (aluminum hyrdroxyde)
               200 mg
               magnesium hydroxide (magnésium hyrdroxyde)
               200 mg
               simethicone (siméticone) 20 mg
   Indication: antacid (antacide)

Extra Strength Mylanta
   Generic/Dose: aluminum hydroxide (aluminum hyrdroxyde)
               400 mg
                magnesium hydroxide (magnésium hyrdroxyde)
               400 mg
                simethicone (siméticone) 20 mg
   Indication: antacid (antacide)

Mylanta Supreme Antacid Liquid
Generic/Dose: calcium carbonate (calcium carbonate) 400 mg
magnesium hydroxide (magnésium hyrdroxyde)
135 mg
Indication: antacid (antacide)

Pepcid Complete
Generic/Dose: famotidine (famotidine)10 mg
calcium carbonate (calcium carbonate) 800 mg
magnesium hydroxide (magnésium hyrdroxyde)
165 mg
Indication: antacid (antacide)

Pepcid AC
Generic/Dose: famotidine (famotidine) 10 mg
Indication: antacid (antacide)

3M Titrulac Antacid
Generic/Dose: calcium carbonate (calcium carbonate) 420 mg
Indication: antacid (antacide)

3M Titrulac Extra Strength Antacid
Generic/Dose: calcium carbonate (calcium carbonate) 750 mg
Indication: antacid (antacide)

3M Titrulac Plus Antacid
Generic/Dose: calcium carbonate (calcium carbonate) 420 mg
simethicone (siméticone) 21 mg
Indication: antacid (antacide)
indigestion (dyspepsie)

Maximum Strength GasAid Softgels
Generic/Dose: simethicone (siméticone) under 25 mg
Indication: gas relief

Imodium A-D Liquid
Generic/Dose: loperamide hydrochloride (lopérimide
chlorhydrate) 1 mg/5 ml
Indication: diarrhea (diarrhée)
elixir (élixir)

Imodium Advanced Chewable Tablets
  Generic/Dose: loperamide hydrochloride (lopérimide
                chlorhydrate) 2 mg
  simethicone   (siméticone) 125 mg
  Indication: diarrhea (diarrhée)

Lactaid Drops
  Generic/Dose: lactase 3000 USP units
  Indication: lactose intolerance

Dulcolax
  Generic/Dose: bisacodyl (bisacodyl) 5 mg tablet
                bisacodyl (bisacodyl) 10 mg/suppository
                (suppositoire)
  Indication: constipation (constipation)
                laxative (laxatif)
Ex-Lax
  Generic/Dose: sennosides (sennosides calciques)15 mg
  Indication: constipation (constipation)
                stimulant laxative (laxatif)

Ex-Lax Gentle Strength with Stool Softener
  Generic/Dose: docusate sodium (docusate sodique) 65 mg
                sennosides (sennosides calciques) 10 mg
  Indication: laxative (laxatif)
                constipation (constipation)

Ex-Lax Milk of Magnesia
  Generic/Dose: magnesium hydroxide (magnésium hyrdroxyde)
                400 mg/5 ml
  Indication: laxative (laxatif)
                constipation (constipation)

Ex-Lax Stool Softener Caplets
  Generic/Dose: docusate sodium (docsate sodique) 100 mg/capsule
  Indication: laxative (laxatif)
                constipation (constipation)

Maalox Antacid and Anti Gas
Generic/Dose: magnesium hydroxide (magnésium hyrdroxyde)
200 mg
aluminum hydroxide (aluminum hyrdroxyde)
200 mg
simethicone (siméticone) 20 mg
Indication: antacid (antacide)
indigestion (dyspepsie)

Maalox Maximum Strength Maalox Antacid/Anti-Gas
Generic/Dose: magnesium hydroxide (magnésium hyrdroxyde)
400 mg
aluminum hydroxide (aluminum hyrdroxyde)
400 mg
simethicone (siméticone) 40 mg
Indication: antacid (antacide)
indigestion (dyspepsie)

Perdiem Overnight Relief Laxative
Generic/Dose: psyllium (psyllium) 3.25 mg
senna (séné) 0.74 g
Indication: laxative (laxatif)
constipation (constipation)

Perdiem Fiber Therapy
Generic/Dose: psyllium (psyllium) 4.03 gm/tsp
Indication: laxative (laxatif)
constipation (constipation)

Anusol Suppositories
Generic/Dose: topical starch (amidon topique) 51%
benyl alcohol (alcool bénylique)
hydrogenated vegetable oil (huile végétale
hydrogénée)
tocopheryl acetate (alpha – tocophérol acetate)
Indication: hemorrhoid (hémorroéde)
suppository (suppositoire)

Anusol HC-1
 Generic/Dose: hydrocortisone (hydrocortisone acetate) 1%
 Indication: hemorrhoid (hémorroéde)
               suppository (suppositoire)

Rolaids
 Generic/Dose: calcium carbonate (calcium carbonate) 550 mg
               magnesium hydroxide (magnésium hyrdroxyde)
               110 mg
 Indication: indigestion (dyspepsie)

Rolaids Extra Strength
 Generic/Dose: calcium carbonate (calcium carbonate) 675 mg
               magnesium hydroxide (magnésium hyrdroxyde)
               135 mg
 Indication: indigestion (dyspepsie)

Tucks
 Generic/Dose: witch hazel (hamamélis) 50% solution
 Indication: hemorrhoid (hémorroéde)

Zantac 75
 Generic/Dose: ranitidine (ranitidine chlorhydrate) 75 mg
 Indication: indigestion (dyspepsie)

Emetrol
 Generic/Dose: dextrose (dextrose) 1.87 g/5 ml
               fructose (fructose) 1.87 g/5 ml
               phosphoric acid (acide phosphorique)
               21.5 mg/5 ml
 Indication: nausea (nausée)
               vomiting (vomissement)

Surfak Liqui-Gels
 Generic/Dose: docusate calcium (docusate sodique) 240 mg
 Indication: laxative (laxatif)
               constipation (constipation)

Metamucil
    Generic/Dose: psyllium (psyllium) 3.4 grams/teaspoon
    Indication: constipation (constipation)
                   laxative (laxatif)

Pepto-Bismol
    Generic/Dose: bismuth subsalicylate (bismuth subgallatum) 262
                       mg/15 ml
                   (contains 130 mg of non-aspirin salicylate)
    Indication: antacid (antacide)

Correctol
    Generic/Dose: bisacodyl (bisacodyl) 5 mg
    Indication: laxative (laxatif)
                   constipation (constipation)

Colace
    Generic/Dose: docusate sodium (docusate sodique) 50 mg
    Indication: constipation (constipation)
                   laxative (laxatif)

Peri-Colace
    Generic/Dose: docusate sodium (docusate sodique) 100 mg
                       casanthrol 30 mg
    Indication: constipation (constipation)
                       laxative (laxatif)

Citrucel Fiber Therapy
    Generic/Dose: methylcellulose (méthylcellulose) 105 mg/gram
    Indication: laxative (laxatif)
                   constipation (constipation)

Gaviscon Regular Strength Antacid Tablets
    Generic/Dose: aluminum hydroxide (aluminum hyrdroxyde)
                       80 mg
                   magnesium trisilicate (magnesium) 20 mg
    Indication: antacid (antacide)

Gaviscon Extra Strength Antacid Tablets
  Generic/Dose: aluminum hydroxide (aluminum hyrdroxyde)
                160 mg
                magnesium carbonate (magnesium) 105 mg
  Indication: antacid (antacide)

Gly-Oxid Liquid (antiseptic oral cleanser)
  Generic/Dose: carbamide peroxide 10% solution
  Indication: oral antiseptic solution

Tagamet HB 200
  Generic/Dose: cimetidine (cimétidine) 200 mg
  Indication: indigestion (dyspepsie)

Tums Regular Strength
  Generic/Dose: calcium carbonate (calcium carbonate) 500 mg
  Indication: indigestion (dyspepsie)

Tums E-X
  Generic/Dose: calcium carbonate (calcium carbonate) 750 mg
  Indication: indigestion (dyspepsie)

Tums Ultra
  Generic/Dose: calcium carbonate (calcium carbonate) 1000 mg
  Indication: indigestion (dyspepsie)

Anbesol (Oral Anesthetic)
  Generic/Dose: benzocaine (benzocaïne) 20% - maximum
                strength gel
                benzocaine (benzocaïne) 7.5% - infant strength
                benzocaine (benzocaïne) 10% - junior strength
  Indication: oral analgesic
                topical medication

Preparation H Cream
  Generic/Dose: petrolatum (petroleum) 18%
                glycerin (glycérine) 12%
                shark liver oil 3%
                phenylephrine hydrochloride (phényléphrine
                  chlorhydrate) 0.25%

Indication: hemorrhoid (hémorro_de)
               topical cream

Preparation H Suppositories
    Generic/Dose: cocoa butter 85.5%
               shark liver oil 3%
               phenylephrine hydrochloride (phényléphrine
               chlorhydrate) 0.25%
    Indication: hemorrhoid (hémorro_de)
               suppository (suppositoire)

Amphojel
    Generic/Dose: aluminum hydroxide (aluminum hyrdroxyde)
               320 mg/5 ml
    Indication: antacid (antacide)

Donnagel
    Generic/Dose: attapulgite (attapulgite de mormoiron activée)
               600 mg/15 ml
    Indication: diarrhea (diarrhée)

Mitrolan
    Generic/Dose: calcium polycarbophil (polycarbophile sel de Ca)
               500 mg
    Indication: constipation (constipation)
               laxative (laxatif)

Female Personal Hygiene

Excedrin Migraine
    Generic/Dose: acetaminophen (paracétamol) 250 mg
               aspirin (acid acétylsalicylique) 250 mg
               caffeine (caféine) 65 mg
    Indication: analgesic (analgésique)

Mycelex-3
    Generic/Dose: butoconazole nitrate (butoconazole nitrate) 2%
    Indication: vaginal yeast infection
               3 day therapy

Mycelex-7
   Generic/Dose: clotrimazole 100 mg/vaginal insert
   Indication: vaginal yeast infection
                   7 day therapy

Gyne-Lotimin 3 Vaginal Cream
   Generic/Dose: clotrimazole 2% 100 mg/applicator
   Indication: vaginal yeast infection
                   3 day treatment
                   vaginal applicator

Massengill Disposable Douche with Poviodone-Iodine
   Generic/Dose: povidone (povidone iodée) vinegar and water
                   solution
   Indication: vaginal antiseptic solution

Maximum Strength Midol Menstrual
   Generic/Dose: acetaminophen (paracétamol) 500 mg
                   caffeine (caffeine) 60 mg
                   pyrilamine maleate (mépyramine maléate) 15 mg
   Indication: analgesic (analgésique)
                   menstruation (menstruation)

Maximum Strength Midol P. M. S.
   Generic/Dose: acetaminophen (paracétamol) 500 mg
                   pamabrom 25 mg
                   pyrilamine maleate (mépyramine maléate) 15 mg
   Indication: menstruation (menstruation)

Maximum Strength Midol Teen
   Generic/Dose: acetaminophen (paracétamol) 500 mg
                   pamabrom 25 mg
   Indication: menstruation (menstruation)

Skin and Hair Care

Bactine Solution
    Generic/Dose: benzalkonium chloride (benzalkonium chlorure)
               0.13%
               lidocaine hydrochloride (lidocaïne chlorhydrate)
               2.5%
    Indication: antiseptic (antiseptique)
                   topical anesthetic

Donboro Astringent Solution
    Generic/Dose: aluminum acetate (aluminium aceticum solution)
               525 mg
    Indication: analgesic (analgésique)
                   minor skin irritations

Tegrin Dandruff Shampoo
    Generic/Dose: coal tar solution (goudron de hoville extrait) 7%
               (USP equivalent to 1.1% coal tar)
    Indication: dandruff (séborrhee sèche)

Tegrin Skin Cream for Psoriasis
    Generic/Dose: 5% coal tar USP (goudron de hoville extrait)
               (= 0.8% coal tar)
    Indication: psoriasis (psoriasis)

Pin-X
    Generic/Dose: pyrantel pamoate (pyrantel emboate) 50 mg/ml
    Indication: pinworm (oxyure)

Nizoral A-D Shampoo
    Generic/Dose: ketoconazole solution (kétoconazole) 1%
    Indication: antifungal

Compound W (Removal of common warts)
    Generic/Dose: 40% salicylic acid (salicylamide)
    Indication: wart (verrue)

Dermoplast Spray - Hospital Strength
  Generic/Dose: benzocaine USP (benzocaïne) 20% (topical
            anesthetic)
          menthol (menthol) 0.5% (antipyretic)
  Indication: relief of itching
          analgesic (analgésique)
          topical medication

Dermoplast Antibacterial Spray-Hospital Strength
  Generic/Dose: benzethonium chloride USP 0.2%
          benzocaine USP (benzocaïne) 20%
          menthol (menthol) 0.5%
  Indication: antibacterial
          topical anesthetic
          relief of itching
          topical medication

Thera-Gesic Topical Therapeutic Analgesic Cream
  Generic/Dose: methyl salicylate (salicylate de méthyl) 15%
            menthol (menthol) 1%
  Indication: topical anesthetic
          topical medication

Desenex
  Generic/Dose: miconazole nitrate (miconazole) 2%
  Indication: antifungal
          ringworm (teigne tonsurante)
          athlete's foot (pied d'athlète)

Lamisil AT Cream 1%
  Generic/Dose: terbinafine hydrochloride (turbinafine
            chlorhydrate) 1%
  Indication: relief of itching
          athlete's foot (pied d'athlète)
          ringworm (teigne tonsurante)

Caladryl Lotion
  Generic/Dose: calamine (calamine) 8% solution

pramoxine hydrochloride (pramocaïne
chlorhydrate) 1% solution
Indication: antipruritic
poison ivy/oak (Rhus toxicodendron)

Cortizone 5
Generic/Dose: hydrocortisone (hydrocortisone acétate) 0.5%
Indication: relief of itching

Cortizone 10
Generic/Dose: hydrocortisone (hydrocortisone acetate) 1.0%
Indication: relief of itching

Neosporin Antibiotic Ointment
Generic/Dose: polymyxin B sulfate (polymysin B sulfate) 5000
    units
bacitracin zinc (bacitracine) 400 units
neomycin (néomycine sulfate) 3.5 mg
Indication: antibiotic (antibiotique)
topical medication

Neosporin with Analgesic Ointment
Generic/Dose: polymyxin B sulfate (polymysin B sulfate) 10,000
    units
neomycin (neomycine sulfate) 3.5 mg
pramoxine hydrochloride (pramocaïne
chlorhydrate) 10 mg
bacitracin zinc (bacitracine) 500 units
Indication: antibiotic (antibiotique)
analgesic (analgésique)
topical medication

Nix Cream Rinse
Generic/Dose: permethrin (perméthrine) 280 mg
Indication: lice (louse)

Polysporin
Generic/Dose: polymyxin B sulfate (polymysin B sulfate) 10,000units

bacitracin zinc (bacitracine) 500 units
Indication: antibiotic (antibiotique)
topical medication

Wart-Off Liquid
Generic/Dose: salicylic acid (salicylamide) 17% solution
Indication: wart (verrue)
topical medication

Cortaid Maximum Strength Cream and Ointment
Generic/Dose: hydrocortisone (hydrocortisone acétate) 1%
Indication: topical medication
anti-pruritic

Betadine First-aid Antibiotic and Moisturizing Ointment
Generic/Dose: polymyxin B sulfate (polymyxine B sulfate) 10,000
IU/gram
bacitracin (bacitracine) zinc 500 IU/gram
Indication: antibiotic (antibiotique)
topical medication

Betadine Ointment
Generic/Dose: povidone (providone iodée) 10% solution
Indication: cleansing solution
topical medication

Lotimin AF Cream
Generic/Dose: clotrimazole cream 1%
Indication: antifungal
athlete's foot (pied d'athlète)
topical medication

Lotimin AF Antifungal
Generic/Dose: miconazole (miconazole) 2%
Indication: antifungal
topical medication

RID Mousse
    Generic/Dose: piperonyl butoxide (pepéronyl butoxyde) 4%
                pyrethrum extract (pyréthrum extrait) (equivalent
                to 0.33% pyrethrines)
    Indication: lice (louse) removal

Zanfel Poison Ivy Cream
    Generic/Dose: polyethylene granules
                sodium lauryl sarcosinate
                nonoxynol-9
                C12-15 pareth-9
                disodium EDTA
                quatemium-15
                carbomer 2%
    Indication: relief of itching
                poison ivy/oak (Rhus toxicodendron)

Maximum Strength RID Lice Killing Shampoo
    Generic/Dose: piperonyl butoxide (pepéronyl butoxyde) 4%
                pyrethrum extract (pyréthrum extrait) (equivalent
                to 0.33% pyrethrines)
    Indication: lice (louse) removal

Miscellaneous Medications

Maximum Strength Nytol
    Generic/Dose: diphenhydramine (diphénhydramine chlorhydrate)
                50 mg
    Indication: insomnia (insomnie)

Simply Sleep
    Generic/Dose: diphenhydramine hydrochloride (diphénhy
                dramine chlorhydrate) 25 mg
    Indication: insomnia (insomnie)

Bonine - Motion Sickness (mal des transports)
    Generic/Dose: meclizine hydrochloride (méclozine chlorhydrate)
                25 mg
    Indication: motion sickness (mal des transports)

Unisom - Insomnia (insomnie)
  Generic/Dose: doxylamine succinate (doxylamine succinate)
                 25 mg
  Indication: insomnia (insomnie)

Sominex Original Formula
  Generic/Dose: diphenhydramine hydrochloride (diphénhy-
                 dramine chlorhydrate) 25 mg
  Indication: sleeping aid

Visine Original
  Generic/Dose: tetrahyrozoline hydrochloride (tétryzoline
                 chlorhydrate) 0.05%
  Indication: temporary relief of eye irritation
                 ophthalmic solution

Dramamine Original
  Generic/Dose: dimenhydrinate (diménhydrinate) 50 mg
  Indication: motion sickness (mal des transports)

Debrox Drops
  Generic/Dose: carbamine peroxide 6.5% solution
  Indication: earwax removal
                 otic solution

Nicoderm CQ Step 1
  Generic/Dose: nicotine (nicotine forme) 21 mg/24 hours
  Indication: smoking cessation
                 transdermal

Nicoderm CQ Step 2
  Generic/Dose: nicotine (nicotine forme) 14 mg/24 hours
  Indication: smoking cessation
                 transdermal

Nicorderm CQ Step 3
  Generic/Dose: nicotine (nicotine forme) 7 mg/24 hours
  Indication: smoking cessation
                 transdermal

Nicorette Mint 4 mg Chewing Gum
   Generic/Dose: nicotine (nicotine forme) 4 mg
   Indication: smoking cessation
                  nicotine gum

Nicorette Mint 2 mg Chewing Gum
   Generic/Dose: nicotine (nicotine forme) 2 mg
   Indication: smoking cessation
                  nicotine gum

Vivarin
   Generic/Dose: caffeine (caféine) 200 mg
   Indication: stimulant

Multivitamins, Iron supplementation, etc.

Fergon Iron Supplement.
   Generic/Dose:
   Indication: mineral supplement
                 iron deficiency deficiency (anémie ferrique)

Probiotica.
   Generic/Dose: lactobacillus (lactobacillus casei var rhamonosus)
   Indication: dietary supplement

Slow Fe Iron Supplement.
   Generic/Dose: ferrous sulfate 160 mg
   Indication: dietary supplement
                 iron deficiency anemia (anémie ferrique)

Slow Fe Iron Supplement with Folic Acid
   Generic/Dose: ferrous sulfate 160 mg
                  folic acid 400 mcg
   Indication: dietary supplement
                 iron deficiency anemia (anémie ferrique)
                 folic acid deficiency

CHILDREN AND YOUNG ADULT MEDICATIONS

Conversions

1 teaspoon = 5 milliliters (ml)
1 tablespoon = 15 milliliters (ml)
1 dropperful = 0.8 milliliters (ml)

Afrin Nasal Decongestant Children's Pump
Generic/Dose: phenyephrine hydrochloride (phényléphrine
chlorhydrate) 0.25%
Indication: decongestant (décongestant)
nasal spray

Benadryl Children's Allergy/Cold Fastmelt
Generic/Dose: diphenhydramine citrate (diphénhydramine citrate)
19 mg
pseudoephedrine hydrochloride (pseudoéphédrine
chlorhydrate) 30 mg
Indication: decongestant (décongestant)
allergy relief

Natruvent Nasal Saline Spray (Pediatric)
Generic/Dose: oxylometazoline hydrochloride (oxymétazoline
chlorhydrate) 0.05%
Indication: decongestant (décongestant)
preservative free

Children's Mylanta Upset Stomach Relief
Generic/Dose: 400 mg calcium carbonate (calcium carbonate)
/5 ml
Indication: antacid (antacide)
pediatric (médecine infantile)
elixir (élixir)

Motrin Children's Cold Oral Suspension
Generic/Dose: ibuprofen (ibuproféne) 100 mg/5 ml (1 teaspoon)
Indication: analgesic (analgésique)

          pediatric (médecine infantile)
          elixir (élixir)

Motrin Junior Strength Caplets
    Generic/Dose: ibuprofen (ibuproféne) 100 mg
    Indication: analgesic (analgésique)
                 pediatric (médecine infantile)

Tylenol Children's Allergy D Liquid
    Generic/Dose: acetaminophen (paracétamol) 160 mg/5 ml
                 diphenhydramine hydrochloride (diphénhydramine
                    chlorhydrate) 12.5 mg/5 ml
                 pseudoephedrine hydrochloride (pseudoéphédrine
                    chlorhydrate) 15 mg/5 ml
    Indication: analgesic (analgésique)
                 decongestant (décongestant)
                 alcohol free
                 pediatric (médecine infantile)

Tylenol Children's Suspension Liquid
    Generic/Dose: acetaminophen (paracétamol) 160 mg/5 ml
                 (1 teaspoon)
    Indication: analgesic (analgésique)
                 pediatric (médecine infantile)
                 elixir (élixir)

Tylenol Children's Cold Suspension and Chewable Tablets
    Generic/Dose: acetaminophen (paracétamol) 160 mg/5 ml
                 chlorpheniramine maleate (chlorphénanamine
                    maleáte) 1 mg/5 ml pseudoephedrine hydrochlo-
                    ride (pséudoephédrine chlorhydrate) 15 mg/5 ml
    Indication: analgesic (analgésique)
                 pediatric (médecine infantile)

Tylenol Children's Cold Plus Cough Suspension Liquid
    Generic/Dose: acetaminophen (paracétamol) 160 mg/5 ml
                 chlorpheniramine maleate (chlorphénanamine
                    maleáte) 1 mg/5 ml

Indication: dextromethorphan hydrobromide (dextrométhorphane bromhydrate) 5 mg/5 ml
pseudoephedrine hydrochloride (pséudoephédrine
chlorhydrate) 15 mg/5 ml
analgesic (analgésique)
antitussive (expectorant)
pediatric (médecine infantile)
elixir (élixir)

Tylenol Children's Cold Plus Cough Chewable Tablets
Generic/Dose: acetaminophen (paracétamol) 80 mg
chlorpheniramine maleate (chlorphénanamine
maleáte) 0.5 mg
dextromethorphan hydrobromide
(dextrométhorphane bromhydrate) 2.5 mgs
pseudoephedrine hydrochloride (pséudoephédrine
chlorhydrate) 7.5 mgs
Indication: analgesic (analgésique)
antitussive (expectorant)
pediatric (médecine infantile)

Tylenol Children's Flu Suspension Liquid
Generic/Dose: acetaminophen (paracétamol) 160 mg/5 ml
chlorpheniramine maleate (chlorphénanamine
maleáte) 1 mg/5 ml
dextromethorphan hydrobromide
(dextrométhorphane bromhydrate) 7.5 mg/5 ml
pseudoephedrine hydrochloride (pséudoephédrine
chlorhydrate) 15 mg/5 ml
Indication: analgesic (analgésique)
decongestant (décongestant)
pediatric (médecine infantile)

Tylenol Children's Sinus Liquid
Generic/Dose: acetaminophen (paracétamol) 160 mg/5 ml
pseudoephedrine hydrochloride (pséudoephédrine
chlorhydrate) 15 mg/5 ml

Indication: analgesic (analgésique)
                decongestant (décongestant)
                pediatric (médecine infantile)

Benylin Pediatric Cough Suppressant
  Generic/Dose: dextromethorphan hydrobromide
                (dextrométhorphane bromhydrate) 7.5 mg/5 ml
  Indication: antitussive (expectorant)
                elixir (élixir)
                pediatric (médecine infantile)

PediaCare Cough and Cold Liquid
  Generic/Dose: pseudoephedrine hydrochloride (pseudoéphédrine
                chlorhydrate) 15 mg/5 ml
                chlorpheniramine maleate (chlorphenanamine
                maleate) 1 mg/5 ml
                dextromethorphan hydrobromide
                (dextrométhorphane bromhydrate) 5 mg/5 ml
  Indication: antitussive (expectorant)
                decongestant (décongestant)
                elixir (élixir)
                pediatric (médecine infantile)

PediaCare Night Rest Cough and Cold Liquid
  Generic/Dose: pseudoephedrine hydrochloride (pseudoéphédrine
                chlorhydrate) 15 mg/5 ml
                chlorpheniramine maleate (chlorphenanamine
                maleate) 1 mg/5 ml
                dextromethorphan hydrobromide
                (dextrométhorphane bromhydrate) 7.5 mg/5 ml
  Indication: decongestant (décongestant)
                antitussive (expectorant)
                elixir (élixir)
                pediatric (médecine infantile)

Vicks Children's Nyquil
  Generic/Dose: chlorpheniramine maleate (chlorphénanamine
                maleáte) 2 mg/15ml

272 — GLOBETROTTER'S POCKET DOC

dextromethorphan hydrobromide
(dextrométhorphane hydrobromide) 15 mg/15ml
pseudoephedrine HCL (pseudoéphédrine
chlorhydrate) 30 mg/15ml
Indication: decongestant (décongestant)
antitussive (expectorant)
elixir (élixir)
pediatric (médecine infantile)

Pediatric Vicks 44
Generic/Dose: dextromethorphan (dextrométhorphane) under
bromide 10 mg/50 ml
guaifenesin (guaïfénésine) 100 mg/15 ml
Indication: decongestant (décongestant)
elixir (élixir)
pediatric (médecine infantile)

Advil Children's Strength
Generic/Dose: ibuprofen (ibuproféne) 100 mg/5 ml
Indication: analgesic (analgésique)
elixir (élixir)
pediatric (médecine infantile)

Advil Junior Strength Tablets
Generic/Dose: ibuprofen (ibuproféne) 100 mg
Indication: analgesic (analgésique)
pediatric (médecine infantile)

Robitussin Pediatric Strength Cough Suppressant
Generic/Dose: dextromethorphan hydrobromide
(dextromethorphane bromhydrate) 7.5 mg/5 ml
Indication: antitussive (expectorant)
elixir (élixir)
pediatric (médecine infantile)

Robitussin Pediatric Strength Cough & Cold
Generic/Dose: dextromethorphan hydrobromide

(dextromethorphane bromhydrate) 7.5 mg/5 ml
pseudoephedrine hydrochloride (pseudoéphédrine
chlorhydrate) 15 mg/5 ml

Indication: decongestant (décongestant)
antitussive (expectorant)
elixir (élixir)
pediatric (médecine infantile)

INFANT MEDICATIONS

Colds, Gas, Diaper Rash, Skin Conditions

Infant's Mylicon Drops
  Generic/Dose: simethicone (siméticone) 30 mg/0.3 ml
  Indication: gas relief
                 elixir (élixir)
                 infant (nourrison)

A and D Ointment with Zinc Oxide
  Generic/Dose: dimethicone (diméticone) 1%
                 zinc oxide (zinc oxyde) 10%
  Indication: diaper rash
                 infant (nourrison)

Balmex Diaper Rash Ointment
  Generic/Dose: cornstarch 86.9%
                 zinc oxide (zinc oxyde) 10.0%
  Indication: diaper rash
                 infant (nourrison)

Balmex Diaper Rash Ointment
  Generic/Dose: zinc oxide (zinc oxyde) 11.3%
                 Aloe (aloe)
                 Vitamin E (alpha tocophérol acetate)
  Indication: diaper rash
                 infant (nourrison)

Motrin Infants Concentrated Drops
  Generic/Dose: ibuprofen (ibuproféne) 50 mg/1.25 ml
                 (one dropperful)
  Indication: analgesic (analgésique)
                 elixir (élixir)
                 infant (nourrison)

Tylenol Infant's Cold Decongestant and Fever Reducer
Concentrated Drops
  Generic/Dose: acetaminophen (paracétamol) 160 mg/1.6 ml

(2 dropper full)
pseudoephedrine hydrochloride (pséudoephédrine chlorhydrate) 15 mg/1.6 ml (2 dropper full)

Indication: analgesic (analgésique)
decongestant (décongestant)
elixir (élixir)
alcohol free
infant (nourrison)

Tylenol Infant's Cold Decongestant and Fever Reducer
Concentrated Drops plus Cough
    Generic/Dose: acetaminophen (paracétamol) 160 mg/1.6 ml
dextromethorphan hydrobromide (dextrométhor phane bromhydrate) 5 mg/1.6 ml
pseudoephedrine hydrochloride (pséudoephédrine chlorhydrate) 15 mg/1.6 ml

Indication: analgesic (analgésique)
decongestant (décongestant)
elixir (élixir)
infant (nourrison)

Tylenol Infants Concentrated Drops (alcohol free)
    Generic/Dose: acetaminophen (paracétamol) 160 mg/1.6 ml (two droppers full)

Indication: analgesic (analgésique)
elixir (élixir)
infant (nourrison)

Desitin Creamy With Aloe and Vitamin E
    Generic/Dose: zinc oxide (zinc oxyde) 10%
aloe (aloe)
Vitamin E (vitamin E = alpha: tocophérol acetate)

Indication: skin protection
infant (nourrison)

Desitin Regular Ointment
    Generic/Dose: zinc oxide (zinc oxyde) 10%
    Indication: skin protection

diaper rash
infant (nourrison)

Advil Infant's Strength
   Generic/Dose: ibuprofen (ibuproféne) 50 mg/1.25 ml
   Indication: analgesic (analgésique)
                 elixir (élixir)
                 infant (nourrison)

Dimetapp Infant Drops
   Generic/Dose: pseudoephedrine hydrochloride (pseudoéphédrine
                 chlorhydrate) 7.5 mg/0.8 ml
   Indication: decongestant (décongestant)
                 elixir (élixir)
                 infant (nourrison)

Dimetapp Infant Drops Decongestant Plus Cough
   Generic/Dose: pseudoephedrine hydrochloride (pseudoéphédrine
                 chlorhydrate) 7.5 mg/0.8 ml
                 dextromethorphan hydrobromide
                 (dextrométhorphane bromhydrate) 2.5 mg/0.8 ml
   Indication: decongestant (décongestant)
                 antitussive (expectorant)
                 elixir (élixir)
                 infant (nourrison)

Robitussin Cough & Cold Infant Drops
   Generic/Dose: guaifenesin (guaïfénésine) 100 mg/2.5 ml
                 pseudoephedrine HCl (pseudoéphédrine
                 chlorhydrate) 15 mg/2.5 ml
                 dextromethorphan HBr (dextromethorphane
                 bromhydrate) 5 mg/2.5 ml
   Indication: antitussive (expectorant)
                 expectorant (expectorant)
                 elixir (élixir)
                 infant (nourrison)

Robitussin DM Infant Drops
   Generic/Dose: dextromethorphan hydrobromide

(dextromethorphane bromhydrate) 5 mg/2.5 ml
guaifenesin (guaïfénésine) 100 mg/2.5 ml

Indication: decongestant (décongestant)
antitussive (expectorant)
elixir (élixir)
infant (nourrison)

GENERAL OUTPATIENT INSTRUCTIONS

Corneal Abrasion

Corneal abrasions are scratches on the cornea of the eye. The cornea is the clear portion of the eye. Scratches usually result from foreign objects. The evaluation of the eye should be carried out by a physician.

If the eye has been dilated or a patch placed to protect the eye, do not drive a car. Follow up with your ophthalmologist or primary care physician upon returning home.

During the eye examination, pain relief is usually accomplished with a topical medication which completely relieves the pain from a corneal abrasion. However, continued use of this topical medication can result in delayed healing of the abrasion. For this reason, topical drops are usually not prescribed for prolonged use. Oral pain medications can be used for adequate control of pain while the eye heals.

Indications for Physician Consultation
• Prolonged pain refractory to oral pain medications.
• Drainage from the eye.
• Blurred vision.
• Diminished vision.

Croup

Croup is a combination of infection and the inflammation associated with infection and swelling (edema). The edema is a natural response to infection. Edema occurs in virtually all infectious processes. The edema involved with croup involves the voice box (also called the larynx). In this case, croup is associated with a cold.

Clinical symptoms associated with croup are a barking type of cough and, occasionally, difficulty breathing. The symptoms usually worsen at night but resolve within five to seven days.

Acute Attack
• Remain calm so as to keep your child calm. Worsening of the shortness of breath and difficulty breathing may be exacerbated by the child's anxiety.
• Put the child in a hot steamy room. This can be done by using

the bathroom's hot shower or filling a tub full of hot water.
- Improvement in breathing within 10-20 minutes is usually accomplished. After your child has had improvement in breathing, try using a cool humidifier in the child's room.
- Returning to a hot misty atmosphere is also helpful should difficulty breathing recur.
- Make sure the child rests.
- Ensure adequate hydration by using water, juice, tea, or soda.
- Do not feed a child solid food during an acute attack.

Indications for Physician Consultation
- The child's breathing has not significantly improved after 20 minutes in a hot misty atmosphere.
- The child is unable to maintain adequate hydration. This is usually characterized by increased thirst, decreased urine output, listlessness and malaise. Dizziness may also occur.
- The cough persists for more than 5 days.
- Your child is having difficulty swallowing water or saliva.
- The lips or fingers turn blue.
- Your child has increased respiratory rate of greater than 50 per minute.

Dehydration

Dehydration can be severe or mild. Mild dehydration can be replaced with fluids and electrolytes. Drink fluids in small sips. Dietary intake of salt should help replace sodium.

Prevention of dehydration is a primary goal in hot weather, at times of extreme physical activity, or with a high fever. Do not wait until symptoms of dehydration occur. Drink fluids consistently throughout the day.

Symptoms of dehydration include:
- flushed face
- dry, warm skin
- headache
- dry mouth
- thick saliva
- weakness

- cramps in the arms or legs
- confusion
- fatigue or lethargy

If you have noticed that you have dizziness or have had an episode of passing out (syncope) you should seek medical assistance. These complaints reflect more advanced dehydration which may need intravenous fluid replacement and evaluation of electrolytes by measuring blood chemistries.

Sports drinks contain fluids, electrolytes, and glucose. These drinks are readily available sources of electrolytes and glucose. These solutions are rapidly absorbed and may be of great assistance. Most solutions which are readily available are not able to replete all the lost electrolytes and fluids. Nevertheless, when dehydration occurs it is important to drinks fluids.

Should a more balanced solution be required or prescribed, an oral rehydration solution (ORS) can be easily made by any traveler.

Oral rehydration solutions can be made from readily available foods. ORS is absorbed in the proximal small intestine. This makes them very useful in patients with vomiting and/or diarrhea. Be sure to use boiled water or water that is known to be free of any infectious bacteria or parasites. Into one quart of water, add:

2 tablespoons of sugar (other sources of glucose such as honey are
   acceptable)
DO NOT USE ARTIFICIAL SWEETNERS
1/4 teaspoon of salt
1/4 teaspoon of baking soda (bicarbonate of soda)

If baking soda is not available, add some orange juice and another 1/4 teaspoon of salt. This will supply some potassium. Bananas are also a good source of potassium.

Drink the solution in small sips. Drink frequently. One way of assessing the level of hydration is the frequency and color of urination. If the urine is a dark yellow and is present in only small volumes, dehydration is likely. Urine that has a normal yellow color and urination that occurs four to five times per day reflects normal intravascular volume.

When vomiting and diarrhea are present, follow the instructions in those specific sections. Remember, the ORS solution, when taken frequently in small amounts, will not make diarrhea worse. When vomiting is present, small sips are important. Some solution will be absorbed during vomiting.

Diarrhea and Vomiting in the Adult

Diarrhea and vomiting are extremely common ailments when traveling in foreign countries. The two may be coexistent or separate complaints. In most cases, diarrhea is self-limited and is likely due to food poisoning. The goals of outpatient care are to ensure adequate hydration while the acute illness resolves. The best approach for managing these problems is to direct therapy at the two problems separately. Read the following thoroughly prior to instituting any treatment.

Diarrhea
- Do not take milk or milk products.
- Avoid tea and coffee. These contain caffeine which increase urination, small bowel fluid, and electrolyte secretion.
- Juices may be tolerated but may also exacerbate the problem since metabolism of carbohydrates (fructose) may be diminished during acute infectious (either viral or bacterial) diarrhea. Try some juices but be wary.
- Use clear liquids with simple carbohydrates (glucose) as these are usually easily absorbed within the small intestine. Other alternatives are Jello, popsicles, flat ginger ale. Products such as Gatorade, if available, are also useful.

Oral rehydration solutions (ORS) as recommended by the World Health Organization (WHO) can easily be made by travelers. See the previous section on Dehydration for instructions on preparing and using an oral rehydration solution.

If you are also experiencing vomiting, take small sips of liquids. These are better tolerated than large volumes.

The first 24 hours are important for maintaining normal hydration. If the diarrhea improves over the next 24 to 48 hours, you may begin to slowly increase the food. Again, avoid milk or milk products. Yogurt, which may have a low lactose content, can be attempted.

Always wash your hands when using the bathroom so that others may not be afflicted.

Indications for Physician Consultation
- Diarrhea which persists after 3 or 4 days needs further evaluation.
- Dehydration
- Change in mental status
- Bloody diarrhea should be evaluated immediately.

Vomiting
Drink clear liquids only. These should be administered in small amounts until the patient is able to drink adequately.

Watch closely for aspiration of fluids. This is usually present when a patient begins to cough during drinking. If the patient develops a cough after drinking fluid or becomes short of breath, aspiration may have occurred. In this event, patients should seek medical advice.

Return to a normal diet 12 hours after vomiting ceases. The diet should consist of bland foods.

Indications for Physician Consultation
- Vomiting of bright red blood
- Vomiting of material which appears to have coffee grounds present
- Vomiting for more than 24 hours, especially if other chronic medical problems are present
- Dehydration
- Change in mental status
- Fever

Head Injury
Any head injury can be serious. If loss of consciousness has occurred, medical evaluation is mandatory. The following instructions are useful for patients who have been evaluated by a physician. They do not supplant the instructions provided by the physician or the medical staff. These are intended to assist you in providing care to a patient who may have had a potentially serious head injury.

Observe the patient carefully over the next 24 hours.

Headache

It is not uncommon to have a headache after a head injury. Ice packs placed on the injured area for 20 to 30 minutes may be helpful. The patient may take acetaminophen or ibuprofen for pain. No other medications should be taken unless approved by a physician.

Nausea and Vomiting

Nausea and limited vomiting (one or two episodes) are not unusual after a head injury. If these complaints persist or if they increase in their severity or frequency, re-evaluation by the physician is recommended.

Drowsiness or Dizziness

Head injury patients frequently experience these complaints. Close observation of the patient during the day is recommended. At night, the patient should be wakened every four hours to check his or her level of consciousness. Observe whether or not it is easy to awaken the patient. Ask the patient simple, direct questions such as: Where are you? What day is it? What is your birthday? The patient's answers will help you evaluate his/her mental status.

Nutrition

Clear liquids are recommended for 24 hours. Vomiting may exist. In this case, small sips of fluids are best. Watch for aspiration of liquids.

Indications for Physician Consultation

Contact your physician, either before or after an evaluation, should any of the following occur:
- There is blood or clear fluid draining from the nose or ears
- Stumbling, difficulty walking, or signs of diminished coordination
- Changes in patient's mental status
- Convulsions or seizures
- Slurred speech or difficulty speaking
- Weakness in any part of the body, including the face
- Inability to fully arouse the patient
- Confusion
- Increased headache, nausea, or vomiting

- Changes in vision such as blurred vision, double vision, flashing lights or decreased peripheral vision

Nosebleed

Nosebleeds may be managed without direct professional intervention. If bleeding persists, professional treatment may be best.

To stop a nosebleed:
- Sit up. Do not lie down.
- Blow the nose free of clots.
- Pinch the lower half of the nose between the thumb and index finger. Try to compress as much of the soft portion of the lower nose as possible.
- Maintain the "pinch" for 10 minutes.
- If the bleeding continues after 10 minutes of compression, seek medical assistance.

General Instructions after Professional Intervention

It is likely that your physician placed a packing within the nose or applied cautery to the bleeding vessel.
- Avoid blowing your nose with great force.
- Avoid medications such as aspirin, ibuprofen, Motrin, Advil, etc. These medications decrease the ability of platelets to form a clot at the site of bleeding. The primary function of platelets is to control bleeding.
- Avoid heavy lifting or bending over. These maneuvers may increase the pressure within the nose.
- If you sneeze, open your mouth and sneeze through your mouth. This will reduce the pressure within the nose.
- Avoid drinking excessively hot beverages. This has been associated with recurrence of bleeding.

Otitis Media (Ear Infection)

Otitis media is an infection of the middle ear. The middle ear is located behind the eardrum. Otitis media frequently occurs during or shortly after a cold. It is during these events when bacteria travel through the eustachian tube and infect the sterile fluid behind the eardrum. Most ear infections occur in children. They are less common in adults.

Usually otitis media requires medical treatment with antibiotics. This avoids potential complications such as hearing loss.

Signs and symptoms indicating that an otitis media may be present are:
- Fever
- Earache and/or ear pressure
- Decreased hearing
- Nausea and/or vomiting
- Fluid draining from the ear
- Decreased appetite
- Irritability

After you have been evaluated by a physician, antibiotics are usually prescribed. Take these medications as directed by your physician. Most antibiotic regimens are for 10 days. Some courses of antibiotics may extend to 14 days.
- Follow the instructions for the antibiotics.
- Acetaminophen may be used for pain relief.
- Do not place anything in the ear.
- Have the patient re-evaluated in 10 to 14 days to insure that the infection has been eradicated.

Re-evaluation by a physician should be done if:
- Symptoms do not improve within two days.
- Fever does not improve.
- The pain worsens or there is an onset of vomiting.
- The patient appears too ill for the situation.

Diarrhea and Vomiting: Infants and Children
Vomiting and diarrhea are commonly associated problems. Children should be evaluated by a physician. The following are general recommendations from the American College of Pediatrics regarding supportive care for these patients.

Diarrhea
Give clear liquids for the first 4 to 6 hours. This should be a glucose-electrolyte containing solution such as:

- popsicles
- Gatorade
- Pedialyte
- liquid cherry jello
- Oral Rehydration Solution (ORS). Refer to Dehydration Section.

After 6 to 8 hours of providing clear liquids, slowly advance the child's diet.

- For infants, mix the formula with twice as much water. This will dilute the formula to half strength. Administer for next 24 hours.
- If mother is breast feeding, give clear liquids for two feedings, then restart breast feeding.
- Older children may start with bland items like bananas, rice, toast, applesauce, tea, crackers, clear soups or broths, and other high-carbohydrate foods.
- Avoid dairy products for 24 hours.

Vomiting

- Give clear liquids for 4 to 6 hours, as described above.
- Start infants with 1/2 to one ounce of fluids every 30 minutes. If the child is able to drink from a cup, offer 1 to 2 teaspoons of fluid every 10 to 15 minutes. Increase as tolerated but watch closely.
- If the child begins to vomit, stop administering fluids for about one hour and then restart.
- If the vomiting has stopped or improved over the next 6 hours, advance the child's diet gradually.

Indications for Physician Consultation

- Vomiting or diarrhea increases in frequency, volume or severity.
- Diarrhea or vomiting occurs for more than 24 hours.
- Signs of dehydration occur. These include:
  Mental status changes
  Dry mouth
  Decreased urine output
  Weight loss
  High fever

Fever: Children Under the Age of Six

Fever is usually associated with infection from either a bacteria or virus. If the rectal or ear temperature is greater than 100 degrees Fahrenheit, it should be treated to provide comfort and prevent febrile seizures.

Always keep track of the temperature. This is often useful should further evaluation of the child be required.

Fever reduction can be accomplished by:
- dressing the child in lightweight clothing.
- providing plenty of cool fluids.
- giving sponge baths with tepid water for 15 minutes every hour.
- giving acetaminophen in pediatric doses.

Note: Avoid aspirin and salicylate containing medications due to the possibility of Reyes syndrome.

Sprains and Contusions

Sprains are injuries to ligaments. Ligaments are tissues which connect two different sets of tissues. Contusions are large bruises.

General instructions
- Immobilize the injured area with a bandage or brace.
- Elevate the injured area above the level of the heart whenever possible. This maneuver helps to reduce the swelling. It is most effective during the first 48 hours.
- During the first 48 hours after the injury, cold packs can assist in reducing the swelling. Apply the packs for 20 to 30 minutes every two hours as needed.
- After the first 48 hours, moist heat applied for 20 to 30 minutes every two hours improves the healing of the injured area.
- Rest the joint as much as possible. Do not participate in activities which may re-injure the area.

Urinary Tract Infection

Urinary tract infections are common in adults. Symptoms of a urinary tract infection are painful urination, frequent urination, urination at night, and urination of small volumes. Urinary Tract Infections (UTI) are usually treated with a 10- to 14-day course of antibiotics.

After you have been evaluated:
- Take your antibiotics as directed.
- If you have pain or fever, 1 or 2 tablets of acetaminophen or aspirin may be taken every 4 to 6 hours.
- If your symptoms have not improved within 48 hours, contact your physician.
- Drink plenty of fluids, about 8 to 10 eight-ounce glasses per day.

AMERICAN EMBASSIES AND CONSULATES

The American presence in a foreign country varies depending upon the size of the country and various other factors outside the realm of healthcare. The diplomatic mission to a country is basically divided into the Embassy, usually located in the capital city, regional Consulates, and American Presence Post (APP). The APP's primary mission is to be one of business support. Assistance for medical affairs would best be fulfilled by contacting the Embassy or Consulate. All offices are closed on French and American Holidays.

In France, the American Embassy is in Paris. Consulates are located in Marseille and Strasbourg. After hours emergency calls are usually referred to the Embassy in Paris.

Embassies and Consulates usually have a list of physicians who may assist you. As always, use this book to its fullest. The treating physician may or may not have an excellent understanding of English.

American Embassy France

Address: 2 Avenue Gabriel, 75008 Paris, France
Telephone: (33) 1 43 12 22 22
Fax: (33) 1 42 66 97 83
Web site: www.amb-usa.fr

American Consulates France
Consulat General des Etats-Unis-d'Amerique

Marseille
Address: Place Varian Fry, 13006 Marseille, France

Mailing Address: Place Varian Fry, 13286 Marseille, France, Cedex 6

Open Monday-Friday
09:00-12:00 & 14:00-17:00

Telephone: (33) 4 91 55 09 07
Fax: (33) 4 91 55 09 47

Strasbourg
Office/Mailing Address:15, Avenue d'Alsace, 67802 Strasbourg

Office Hours:
Monday Through Friday
09:00-13:00 & 14:00-17:00

Telephone: (33) 3 88 35 31 04
Fax: (33) 3 88 24 06 95

INDEX

Quick Order Form

Online orders: http://www.pktdoc.com

Online orders receive a 20% discount. Same as Amazon.com

Fax orders: 303-684-8765

Postal orders: Caduceus International, LLC
                  P.O. Box 144
                  Hygiene, CO 80533

Item	Price	Quantity	Total
Globetrotter's Pocket Doc	$34.95 x	_____	= $_____
Subtotal			= $ _____
Shipping and handling: $ 4.00 / book			
Colorado residents please add 7% for sales tax. (online sales tax is calculated only if the internet site and the ship to address are in the same state.)			= $_____
Total:			= $ _____

Expedited Shipping available only Online at "www.pktdoc.com

Method of Payment:

❑ Money Order

(Money Orders Made Out to Caduceus International, LLC)

❑ MasterCard   ❑ VISA

Credit Card Information:

Card number: __ __ __ __ __ __ __ __ __ __ __ __ __ __ __ __

_____   _____

Expiration Date   Authorized Signature (as shown on credit card)

Name: _____

Address: _____

City: _____ State: _____ Zip:_____

Daytime phone: (   ) _____Email: _____

Caduceus International, LLC will not to release any information to third parties.

Printed in the United States
20774LVS00004B/49-102